A Call to Mind

A Call to Mind

A Story of Undiagnosed Childhood
Traumatic Brain Injury

Claire Galloway

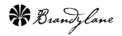

Printed in the United States

ISBN: 978-1-9399309-4-1

LCCN: 2017950791

Published by

🌸 *Brandylane* Publishers, Inc.
WWW.BRANDYLANEPUBLISHERS.COM

For you, Luke. For Good.

"All types of traumatic brain injury, inside and outside sports, can cause permanent or progressive neuropsychiatric illnesses, and because they are neuropsychiatric illnesses, we as a society have failed to recognize their seriousness and broad prevalence, and we have failed to uplift and empathize with the sufferers like we would have if these illnesses were physical illnesses. It is high time we did something collectively as a modern society in tackling chronic traumatic encephalopathy and post-traumatic encephalopathy, in all forms, especially in children."

—Bennett Omalu, MD, MBA, MPH, CPE, DAPB-AP, CP, FP, NP

Foreword

This is a story that encapsulates how ignorance can result in tragedy. Claire Galloway's son Luke was two years old when he was hit in the head by a swing while at the playground. His mother soon noticed changes in his behavior, as a formerly sunny child became anxious and clingy. Over time his challenges increased as he experienced undiagnosed seizures, periods of agitation, difficulties expressing himself, and severe depression. The first act of ignorance occurred soon after the injury, when Luke's pediatrician told his mother not to take him to an emergency room (ER) because he had not lost consciousness. However, loss of consciousness is not a necessary element in diagnosing concussion or mild brain injury. Instead, the blow to the head, accompanied by changes in Luke's behavior, should have triggered advice to take him to the ER, to determine the nature and extent of the injury. There Luke would have received a neurological examination and possibly a CT scan of the head. While it is likely that CT imaging would have been normal, the absence of an abnormal image does not mean the absence of an injury, as most mild brain injuries are not visible with CT. Thus, the pediatrician's advice was the first in a long chain of wrong-headed information provided to the Galloways by medical professionals and educators. This chain of ignorant advice ultimately resulted in Luke's premature death. Indeed, when as an adolescent Luke was finally diagnosed with a brain injury by a neurologist, the family was told that nothing could be done to help Luke because too long a period of time had elapsed since the onset of his injury—more bad advice.

Luke's story is not unique. Every week I receive emails and calls from parents who are struggling to get the brain injury their child sustained identified so that their child can get the services needed to facilitate the child's ability to competently function in the classroom and at home. All too often these parents are rebuffed by educators and healthcare providers, who turn a deaf ear to them. The outcome of this lack of understanding and knowledge about TBI is often a cascade of negative events leading to educational and social failure. The evidence for this? TBI has been linked to substance abuse, violence, criminality, homelessness, and suicide.

I met Luke's mother in 2008, after an article had been published in *The Wall Street Journal* on the work my colleagues and I were doing on unidentified TBI and its consequences. She felt that the story of her son captured the challenges faced by parents in trying to get their children diagnosed, the first step in getting treatment, to avoid the path to the negative outcomes that result when the pleas of families are ignored. I feel that this book is a textbook case of all that can go wrong. People with brain injuries need to know the alternatives available to them and their families, to support their learning how to address the emotional, cognitive, and other challenges that arise after injury. I believe, as does Luke's mother, that his story sheds light on the situation of so-called mild brain injury, which can lead to so many challenges that can be treated—when knowledge based on science, replaces ignorance.

Dr. Wayne A. Gordon, Ph.D., ABPP/Cn
Jack Nash Professor
Vice Chair, Department of Rehabilitation Medicine
Icahn School of Medicine at Mount Sinai

Prologue

For sixteen years, my son Luke lived with an undiagnosed brain injury, from toddlerhood past the age of legal adulthood. One day he was a normal, playful little boy, and then, in a sudden accident, his head was struck by a swing at a playground—and the next day and every day thereafter, he was changed. Physically unscathed on the outside, he had, in fact, sustained a traumatic brain injury (TBI)—an injury that remained undiagnosed because the medical and educational professionals we encountered had apparently not received the training necessary to identify it.

With all the press these days about TBI in sports and the military, I had hoped information about brain injuries unrelated to these fields would soon follow, giving other affected families the opportunity for a better outcome than we had. But as yet, that doesn't seem to have occurred. As I write this, I am reeling from a recent conversation with an acquaintance who exclaimed, "Isn't it good that Luke's situation won't be happening to others anymore!" When I asked her to explain her thinking, she said, "There's so much information about brain injury now—it's everywhere!"

Thankfully, awareness about TBI *is* increasing—as it relates to athletes and to soldiers returning from war. Yet information about general childhood brain injury, in spite of its common occurrence and the dreadful statistics surrounding it, remains painfully lacking.

According to the Brain Injury Association, www.biausa.org, TBI is the "leading cause of death and disability in children and adolescents."

These brain injuries have many causes, including playground accidents, participation in sports, falls, motor vehicle crashes, and physical abuse (including domestic violence and shaken baby incidents). Yet in this age of medical discovery and technological advances, failure to identify and/or effectively treat closed-head traumatic brain injury remains all too common. The Centers for Disease Control and Prevention website, www.cdc.gov, cites statistics on known cases of TBI that should give pause even to the most casual observer. Children are listed among those with the highest incidence of injury. Based on stories of people I have encountered since 2008, when I began advocating for increased awareness of TBI in children, consequences to the injured child and to the family trying to maneuver through life without appropriate, targeted help are as devastating now as they were when my son was injured in 1987.

Although Luke's injury impacted his social, behavioral, and educational development, he did not receive the professional help he needed, simply because his injury remained unidentified and untreated. Without help, he faced failure upon failure. Having no other explanation for his inability to succeed, he absorbed the message that he was to blame, and as his vain attempts mounted over so many years, he eventually screamed out his anger and frustration to his father and me. From the time he was little, Luke expressed his desire to succeed, and it was indescribably painful to stand helplessly nearby and watch his valiant efforts fail.

During those sixteen years between injury and diagnosis, the doctors we encountered failed to determine the connection between the blow to Luke's head at the playground and the closed-head injury it caused. His teachers did not recognize Luke's developing cognitive weaknesses as caused by TBI and, along with family and friends, many blamed him for not reaching his potential. They saw him as a behaviorally maladjusted young boy and then man. Some continued to blame him even after the injury was finally identified. They did this not because they were mean-spirited, but because they didn't make the connection between Luke's difficulties and the blow his head had sustained. Instead of manifesting with obvious, well-recognized symptoms the way a broken leg or diabetes would, Luke's brain injury altered his behavior and his ability to process information and social cues normally, leading even medical and educational professionals to reach false conclusions about him.

Luke's injury was finally identified as he approached age nineteen, but by then he had internalized the negative judgments cast upon him over all those years. To make matters worse, identifying the problem was not the same thing as finding a solution. Bolstered with hope at finally receiving a diagnosis, Luke eventually succumbed to despair when a workable, effective treatment plan was not found. Wracked with self-doubt and the sense of being a burden to himself and his family, he had nowhere to turn.

At the age of twenty-two years, three months, and twenty-eight days, in a state of utter hopelessness and deep, chronic depression, Luke lifted a gun to his head where the injury had occurred and ended his misery with a single pull of the trigger.

This was the worst tragedy that could have befallen our small family. I loved (and, of course, continue to love) this boy with all my being. Witnessing the travesty of his life—day after day, month after month, and year after year, watching as he sank like a stone in water—was an unending nightmare. It was patently obvious to me that my little boy was night-and-day different after his head was struck in that playground accident, yet no one believed me. As the years went on and Luke's difficulties not only persisted but worsened, I, too, became the target of blame as an ineffective parent, which only made my attempts to find help more futile.

A week or so after the shock of Luke's death, I saw an advertisement for the play *Wicked* and, drawn to the story line, was overwhelmed with a desire to see it. With no immediate access to the show, I purchased the soundtrack, put the disc in the player, and sat on the floor to listen. This was not soft music that might have soothed me, but I kept listening, determined to follow my instincts. When the CD reached the song "For Good," the lyrics immediately grabbed my attention and my grieving heart. The words told not only Elphaba's story, but also Luke's. Elphaba, born with green skin, startled and dismayed all who saw her, and they cast judgment on her for it. Luke, whose invisible injury created roadblocks to success, was similarly judged.

Since that day, I have taken comfort in these words:

For Good

I've heard it said that people come into our lives for a reason,
Bringing something we must learn,
And we are led to those who help us most to grow, if we let them,
And we help them in return.
Well, I don't know if I believe that's true,
But I know I'm who I am today because I knew you.
You'll be with me, like a handprint on my heart.
Who can say if I've been changed for the better?
But, because I knew you, I have been changed for good.[1]

---

1 "For Good" from the Broadway musical *Wicked*. Music and Lyrics by Stephen Schwartz. Copyright © 2003 Stephen Schwartz. All rights reserved. Used by permission of Grey Dog Music (ASCAP).

Nightmare

Friday, November 10, 2006. 7:08 p.m.

I glanced at my watch. The bridge game would begin soon, and I needed to get dressed and out the door or we wouldn't arrive on time. I had hoped a shower would restore some much-needed energy, but dark exhaustion lingered. The sense of pushing through life was familiar to me, especially lately, but today was somehow far worse. I wanted to go to bed and sleep for days.

Lifting the hairdryer, I made a few quick passes. *Good enough*, I thought, shrugging at my still-damp hair. "Good enough" had become easily acceptable. Reaching for my blouse, I realized the phone was ringing. Strangely, so was the doorbell. I called to my husband Mark, who was watching the evening news at the other end of the house, but he didn't hear me.

Thinking it might be Luke returning my afternoon call, I darted for the phone. Although we'd spoken the night before, I was anxious to check in with him again. Our twenty-two-year-old son's long-undiagnosed brain injury had precluded adulthood for him in many ways, and I worried constantly about his well-being. During our last call, his voice had held an unusual mix of exhaustion and distance combined with more softness and love than I had heard him express in years. It was a conversation that had left me feeling confused and more fearful than usual.

"Mrs. Galloway?" Not Luke; disappointment coursed through me.

"Yes."

"I'm from the county police department. Can you come to your front door, please?"

Thrown into an adrenaline-fueled alert, I called out again to Mark. This time he heard me and headed to the door while I tried to finish dressing. Panic enveloped me. My fingers shook as I buttoned my blouse, and I tripped over the legs of my slacks as I pulled them on. Not for the first time, my brain and body felt suddenly divorced from one another. Luke's injury had led to years of life-sapping worry and fear, but this situation pulsed with a palpable threat I could not yet define. The police were at our doorstep. *Why?* I worked to catch my breath.

As I rounded the corner, I was startled to find not one or two, but four officers standing in our foyer. My thoughts spun, uncontrolled. *There must have been an accident. Where is Luke? He must be at the hospital. Hurry! We need to get to him! Please! Hurry!*

But no one was hurrying. About anything. Instead, the officers proceeded slowly into our living room, guiding us to follow them. They only spoke to ask me to sit down, but I didn't want to sit. I wanted to get to Luke. *Why aren't they helping us?* I felt the impulse to rush for the front door, and turned to do so, but one of the policemen gently touched my arm and asked me again to take a seat.

I realized nothing more would be said until I did as they asked, so I sat on the footstool beside me. The faster they told us, the faster we could get to Luke's side to help him. Mark placed himself on the chair next to me and put his arm on mine, and I sensed his matching fear. One of the officers crouched to eye level and took my hand.

"Do you have a son, Luke Galloway?"

"Yes."

"Is your son Luke Galloway?"

"Yes. Yes."

Then Mark wrapped his arms around my body and looked at the officer, whose uniform bore the word "Chaplain."

"Please," Mark said. "Just tell us."

Again we heard, "Do you have a son, Luke Galloway?" We both nodded.

"I need to tell you that your son is dead."

A Blessed Gift

July 1984.

Seven years of hoping, nine months of joyful planning, and there he was. Perfect in every way.

I stared at this carbon copy of my husband and couldn't help but think we were the luckiest parents in the world. *How could two ordinary people have been blessed by such a beautiful miracle?*

Of course, first thing, I counted those little fingers and toes, and noted the Apgar scores. Once the counts were in order—and they were—I settled into enjoyment of this precious new individual, whom we named Luke William.

Luke's personality was marked by a delightful blend of tranquility and curiosity about the world around him. As he soaked life in, he didn't choose to utter more than a few real words until his second birthday, when he simply began to speak in full sentences. Such was Luke's approach to the world: enjoy, absorb, repeat.

He was also a little charmer, willingly (verging on flirtingly) going to any family member or friend who threw a smile or kind word his way. He'd laugh whenever I sang or danced with him to the music that often filled our home. Taking to music easily, two-year-old Luke climbed up on his dad's knees during church service one Sunday morning and "led" the organist. His arms waved to the rhythm of the piece, bringing smiles to the faces of the congregants around us and, of course, to Mark and me.

The first few years of Luke's life were joy-filled and mostly uneventful. Thoroughly laid-back by nature, he was developing on target with all the standard milestones of childhood. Even on long road trips, he passed the time without complaint, quietly looking out the car window or catching his afternoon nap. Whenever I turned around to check on him and he happened to be awake, he rewarded my glance with his sweet smile.

By the time he was two-and-a-half, Luke graced us with his giggle whenever he sensed a celebration at hand. Christmas that year holds a special place in my memory. When Luke visited the shopping mall Santa, he bounded onto Santa's lap and the two began an animated conversation. Luke's sense of humor delighted the man in the red suit, as did his one and only request: he wanted an orange-and-yellow plastic car, just his size, with a door that opened and a hole in the floor through which his feet could make the car go fast. And nothing else would do. Fortunately, Santa was able to deliver, and a happier boy on Christmas morning would be difficult to find.

Luke's first day of nursery school was scheduled for three weeks after Christmas, and I anticipated being dropped off would be difficult for him. With a couple of tricks up my sleeve at the ready to console my son, we walked hand-in-hand up the church steps and through the large double doors into the playroom. Catching his first glimpse of the children already gathered on the floor, Luke simply unhanded himself and ran to join them. He never even turned around as, dumbstruck, I called after him, "Have fun! I'll be back soon!" I made it to the car just in time before a tear or two welled over. I'd never considered the possibility that I would be the one needing consolation.

A Moment Too Late

The accident occurred just a couple of weeks before Luke's third birthday. We'd decided to make good use of a beautiful summer Saturday by heading to a local swimming lake with an adjoining playground. Upon arriving, Luke began playing in the sand, crouching next to us with his toy dump truck, while Mark and I set out the blankets and chairs. Our backs weren't turned for more than a few seconds, but that was all it took. Standing up, I was startled to see Luke's dump truck, but not Luke. I caught sight of him running toward the nearby playground, and immediately I darted after him, calling out his name. But he didn't seem to hear me.

In those few seconds, we watched as our son made a beeline toward a child on a hard plastic swing in full forward position. Horrified and feeling trapped in slow motion, we saw the swing begin its descent. When Luke was directly behind it, the swing reached full speed and began its backward, upward arc, striking him violently on the right side of his head. The impact delivered such force that Luke was thrown into the air and landed about ten feet away. A deadly hush fell over the bystanders, and my stomach lurched. It took only a second or two to reach him. Mark and I both dropped to the ground and bent over him. His eyes were open and his hands were moving. He didn't seem to realize we were there, but I found relief in the simple fact that he was conscious and able to move. In the few seconds it had taken to run to him, I had been afraid he might be dead.

With panic subsiding, I looked my son over carefully. He didn't seem to have a trace of injury on him. We had witnessed the impact and had heard the crack of the swing against his head. The noise of the collision had been loud enough to silence bystanders, and the force of it strong enough to send Luke flying. Yet his head was not cut open, we couldn't see any swelling or bruising, and he was lying quietly—not even crying. *Why wasn't he crying?* Shaken and confused, we swooped him into our arms and ran for a telephone to call his pediatrician. Luke didn't make a sound, but there was a blank, dull look in his eyes. I shuddered and pushed the buttons on the phone as quickly as my trembling fingers would allow.

The doctor tried to calm me as he instructed us to take Luke home and watch him for twenty-four hours for signs of concussion—sleepiness, nausea, confusion, eyes not equally dilated. I wanted to go immediately to the hospital emergency room, but the doctor dissuaded us. He explained that, because there was no outward sign of injury, the hospital would do nothing for Luke and the experience of sitting in an emergency room would only frighten him more.

We had called the doctor for his professional opinion, so we accepted his advice and took our son home, feeling uneasy but hopeful. I carefully checked Luke for signs of concussion over the next twenty-four hours as instructed, and breathed a huge sigh of relief when there were none—at least by my ability to discern. Although quieter and less hungry than usual, Luke seemed alert, his eyes appeared to be dilated normally, and he wasn't excessively sleepy. At the end of those first twenty-four hours, I began to relax into the assumption that all would be fine.

Unexpected Aftermath

And yet, Luke was changed. In the days, months, and years that followed, the relief I felt at finding no outward signs of concussion was replaced by a sense of confusion.

Suddenly, Luke's little face showed signs of prolonged distress. His brows furrowed, and his eyes took on a wild expression I had never before seen in him.

Suddenly, Luke's easygoing, laid-back personality was replaced with palpable agitation. My previously contented little boy now cried often, expressing an inner turmoil that we did not understand and were unable to ease.

Suddenly, this child who had always seemed to enjoy bedtime became hysterically fearful of being left alone. He clung to my legs as I tried to leave his room after tucking him in at night, and his anxiety only escalated over time. Most nights, he cried himself to sleep in the upstairs hallway, having left his bedroom so he could look through the railing and see Mark and me while we read or watched television on the first floor.

Over those first several days, I would periodically ask Luke if his head hurt, but he'd shake his head "no." Whenever I questioned how he felt, he would run around the room in circles, obviously distressed but offering no words to explain how he was feeling. At less than three years of age, he likely had no words to describe what was happening to him.

All of a sudden, Luke didn't sit still when Mark or I tried to read to him. In fact, he could hardly hold still at all. His disposition changed from one of easy, relaxed participation to frenzied motion seemingly devoid of fun. Every now and then, out of the blue, he would clench his hands into fists and shake them in front of himself for a few seconds. In these moments, his whole body trembled without perceptible cause. His eyebrows remained furrowed much of the time, and he took on the appearance of what I can only describe as an agitated stranger. Almost overnight, I barely knew or recognized my precious son. *What is wrong with my little boy?*

For those first couple of weeks, I tried to soothe Luke through the anxiety and agitation that consumed him, assuming that over time any ill effects from the swing's impact would resolve and he would return to his former self.

I told myself that Luke must have developed a severe headache from his accident, and I waited day after day for the headache to ease. Over the next few weeks, I checked and rechecked Luke's head and scalp for any sign of injury, but I could find none. The only thing I could imagine was that perhaps the swing, or the girl on it, had struck Luke's ear, where it might not cause an outward bruise.

Luke's third birthday arrived two weeks later, and I could hardly wait for his annual checkup with the pediatrician. I had phoned the doctor with my concerns several times during those two weeks, and during this appointment I mentioned again how dramatically and suddenly Luke's personality and behavior had changed. The pediatrician, a well-respected, down-to-earth man, told me the parental fun was just beginning. The "threes," he said with a knowing smile, could be much more challenging than the "twos."

I couldn't believe my ears. He made absolutely no connection between the recent blow to Luke's head and the sudden changes in him that I found so confusing and out of character.

I reminded him that we had never experienced any behavioral difficulties with Luke until he was struck by the swing. "Well," he said with a laugh, "all the more reason why the 'threes' will become interesting!"

"Overnight?" I asked.

"You're a first-time mother; trust me here. There is nothing wrong with Luke."

And that was that. But the pediatrician's quick dismissal of my concerns did nothing to salve my worry. He was the professional, and in theory, I should have felt relieved by his assurances. Yet the internal quietude that exists when all is right with the world eluded me.

Almost overnight, the challenge of effectively handling Luke's new outbursts and irrational mood swings began to erode my sense of parental confidence, so I clung to the hope that this was just what the pediatrician had predicted—a sudden case of the "threes." Mark seemed to share the doctor's belief that our son was healthy and was simply beginning to push age-related behavioral limits. Before, we had easily been on the same parenting page, but now, as if the changes to Luke weren't bad enough, my husband and I were experiencing our first shift into opposing views. I tried hard to pretend that Luke was fine. But Luke wasn't fine.

Autumn arrived, and Luke returned to preschool. The previous May, at our year-end conference, his teacher had spoken of him in glowing terms, describing him as one of her easiest and most likeable students. Two weeks into the fall session, however, this same teacher requested an unscheduled conference, and she began the meeting with a question that threw me.

"What is happening in your home?"

She went on, "What has changed? Luke is showing signs of abuse."

I felt the blood drain from my face. "In what way? What do you mean?" I could barely find the words to form those questions. Confusion and unbridled fear ran through me. Of course we weren't abusing Luke. But would this woman use her professional role as teacher to try to lodge a formal accusation? With lightning speed I processed the whole of the situation and realized she had nothing to go on but her own impressions. There were of course no marks on Luke and no actual signs of abuse. Yet her words stung me harder than any I had experienced in my lifetime, and I trembled to think that anyone could imagine we might harm Luke in any way.

She told me he would become "suddenly aggressive," shaking his fists in the air. When she used the word "agitated," I had no doubt she'd observed the same behaviors that had been worrying me for the past several months.

I swore to her that nothing in our household had changed and that Luke was absolutely not being abused, but she seemed unconvinced. I told her about the accident and about the dramatic changes in Luke that had followed. She raised her eyebrows in a look of mistrust, turned, and walked away. I shuddered. I had never before known someone to doubt the care Mark and I were providing for our son, whom we loved so deeply. It was horrifying. Yet I knew something *was* wrong with Luke. *But what?*

With no sign of our familiar Luke returning, I found another nursery school with more structure. Its teachers claimed they would be able to determine the source of Luke's sudden personality change and help him through it. They also were unsuccessful, however, and there were days when Luke cried and clung so hard to my legs I thought my heart would break. I contemplated removing Luke from nursery school entirely, yet I wanted him to experience the social interactions that are a vital part of a child's development.

We opted to keep Luke enrolled despite the challenges inherent in that decision. On several occasions I remained in the school, out of Luke's sight, trying to see for myself how quickly he could calm himself and rejoin the activities. Instead of being reassured, what I witnessed confirmed my worst fears. At school, just like at home, Luke's face would occasionally and without obvious provocation contort into a grimace, and then he would raise his arms with his hands balled into fists and shake them in midair for a few seconds. Soon, his arms and hands would relax and his expression would lose some of its intensity, although his eyebrows remained slightly furrowed. Watching Luke suffer through these sudden and inexplicable outbursts tore me apart. I was frightened for him, of course, but also for the other children in the room. These were strange and disturbing actions to witness. While reading to Luke or just holding him close beside me, I often felt compelled to reach over and lightly massage his forehead, hoping to soften away the angst I saw there. I wanted Luke to be comfortable, and I wished for a glimpse of the laid-back, easily smiling child who had vanished that summer day months ago. Luke didn't seem to mind my efforts, but neither did they help.

My mother visited us several times a year and, as an intimate but outside observer, she revealed her concerns to me as well. Like me, she was appalled that the nursery school teacher had suggested abuse. She knew Mark and I loved Luke more than life itself. But she did notice something new in our family that I hadn't wanted to mention to her: with Luke's difficulties increasing, my relationship with my husband was showing obvious signs of strain.

As time went by and Luke still did not return to his former sweet self, Mark occasionally told me of his regret that his son wasn't as responsive or playful or well-mannered as other children his age. With no alternative cause for Luke's difficulties readily ascertainable, Mark began to question my competence as a mother. That was a turning point in our lives. Mark's frustration over Luke's lagging skills was understandable, but my heart broke as his concern turned in my direction. As the designated at-home parent, I spent hours every day with our son, so I knew, I absolutely knew, that the changes in him arose from that playground accident. But the injury I knew existed was not visible to the eye and had been denied by a respected pediatrician, and Mark chose to align himself with the doctor.

It was a logical choice for Mark to believe the doctor. I couldn't deny that, but understanding his choice did nothing to lessen my sadness and hurt. I focused my energy on helping our son meet his father's expectations of normalcy, and I tried to make our home a place of comfort for all of us. Those efforts were often ineffective, and every failed attempt left us more frustrated. But I had no idea what else to try.

I found being the object of blame so disconcerting that I've given the situation much thought over the years. And I did begin to make sense of the divide between my husband's reaction and my own.

As a child, I contracted post-viral encephalitis. When the acute phase of the illness passed, precautions were taken for several months afterward to prevent damage from any residual brain swelling. The pediatrician then pronounced me cured, though in reality I wasn't—at least not entirely. I spent the next twenty years with an undiagnosed atrial heart rhythm disturbance that had appeared with the onset of the encephalitis.

During the course of those twenty years, I encountered physicians who simply did not believe me when I described passing out in ballet class or dry heaving after a tennis match. My condition seemed to intrigue new doctors called in for consultations. When they also failed to identify the disorder, they blamed it on "women and emotions" and insinuated that I was overreacting and neurotic, causing my own symptoms in an appeal for attention. It wasn't until a new procedure called "electrophysiological mapping" was invented that my malady was finally diagnosed and understood as the legitimately physical problem it was.

My medical history had opened my eyes to the reality that physicians are limited in their ability to diagnose and treat illness by what they've been taught. Mark had no such experience. Still, understanding the logic behind Mark's decision to believe the doctor instead of me didn't make it hurt any less.

I finally realized that questioning my abilities was a better alternative for him as a father than assigning blame directly to his child. Accepting that there was something fundamentally wrong with his son would have been far more difficult for Mark. I could understand this, and it provided some consolation. But there were still days when, as I felt the sting of blame from the man I loved so much, my basest instincts wanted to scream out in frustration: *What more would you like me to do than what I am already doing?* On more than several occasions, I did exactly that. Being suspected by my husband of failing to provide adequate parenting for our child, whom I loved with all my heart, while continuing to witness problematic behaviors in Luke without any sense of how to help him, was maddening and exhausting.

If head trauma was not the source of our son's problems, then what was? I noticed over time that other children tended to pick up new age-related skills more quickly and with more ease than Luke did, so I watched the techniques their parents used. For the most part, our approaches to parenting were quite similar. Why, then, did Luke require so much more effort, often without the desired result?

I reminded myself that I had had two ideal role models in my own mother and father. Learning from them, I mixed business with pleasure in child-rearing techniques, sometimes calling Luke to me to give him a small task to handle, and other times calling him only to give him a treat and a hug. For the most part, this tactic had worked like a charm for my sister and me, but it wasn't working for Luke. My sister and I had learned to be obedient, to view work with anticipation of the reward that followed, and to even perceive work as a privilege.

In the years after the accident with the swing, Luke seemed to make no such connection. If a chore was clear-cut and easily defined, he handled it well. If, as he grew older, multiple steps of instruction were needed to complete the task, Luke might handle the first step quickly enough, but then wander away before beginning step two. He wasn't defiant; he simply appeared not to realize there was anything more to do. And sometimes just capturing his attention away from his building blocks was inordinately difficult, despite the occasional promise of a cookie as soon as he listened. Luke seemed, in fact, to make no connection between his choices and the reward that either did or did not follow, and I found his failure to connect those dots, even on a rudimentary level, worrisome. That Luke didn't complete a job or remain focused was not intrinsically unusual. But his lack of intent and consistency of failure seemed abnormal. Making the situation even more troubling was his confusion whenever I grew angry with him and expected more from him.

"Please" and "Thank You" requirements were consistently applied to Luke's daily routine, but he had a difficult time catching on. The cause and effect of withholding a treat until those simplest vestiges of politeness were uttered seemed to not register with Luke, and I found that baffling.

A few months before Luke turned four, we vacationed at the beach. We met another couple with a son just a few months older than Luke, and the children hit it off well. During a shared boat ride, the young captain allowed the boys to take turns at the wheel under his guidance. It was joyful to watch the three of them. But then, suddenly and inexplicably, Luke's face grimaced. He took hold of the wheel so tightly that his knuckles whitened, and he refused to let go. His tantrum increased and, although we were able to remove him from the situation, he would not let go of his thoughts.

For the remainder of that week, Luke was fixated on the boat and on wanting to go back to steer it. His preoccupation seemed anything but normal and far exceeded what could be termed "bratty" behavior. Even after we returned home, he continued to talk about the boat, with increasing agitation. I rationalized that Luke might be overly tired, and hoped an earlier bedtime and consistently applied discipline might help. It seemed logical to focus on tightening parental controls, as Luke's behavior was exhausting not only himself but Mark and me as well. I leaned into the advice given by the pediatrician, that Luke's highly intelligent brain needed only to be more effectively channeled and his bad behavior more consistently redirected.

Later that summer, a family with a four-year-old son moved in at the end of our block, and he and Luke played together occasionally. The two were in our house one day when, without observable cause,

Luke grimaced, his hands closed into fists, and his arms began to shake. Although the episode was over within seconds, it naturally startled our young guest, as it did me every time I witnessed it. I called the boy's mother to explain, and she surprised me by saying that it had happened several times at her house also. She was a nurse and suggested it might have a physiological, rather than psychological, basis. I overrode concerns and sought counsel once again from the pediatrician, but he only reiterated his position that Luke was a very bright and imaginative little boy, and I should not worry. But I did worry. I worried a lot.

For Luke's fourth birthday, we drove six hours to my mother's home, and the following afternoon, we celebrated with a family picnic and party. The house was filled with people whom Luke did not yet know, and the mood was festive. A colorfully decorated cake shaped like a toy train sat in the center of the dining table, surrounded by deli platters, rolls, and salads. Green-and-blue streamers hung from the chandelier, and a "Happy Birthday" banner was stretched across the wall. Luke took it all in for a few minutes, and then he simply walked up the stairs and put himself to bed.

After the accident, any activity involving an abundance of sensory stimulation caused him to retreat. Gone was his eagerness and excitement in the midst of Christmas preparations; instead, he shied away from them, and he even had to be encouraged to make a "Santa List." For years after the accident, Mark and I would wait in anticipation on Christmas mornings for Luke's footsteps, and for the glee that had blanketed him on Christmas morning at age two-and-a-half. But that never again materialized. Eventually, Mark would go into Luke's bedroom. Without a word, he would lift his already-awake son into his arms and carry him out to the tree, aglow with lights and heaped with packages at its base. Instead of wanting to investigate his gifts, Luke only buried his head in his dad's shoulder.

Halloween was also uncomfortable for him, with its costumes and decorations and ringing doorbells. I tried to override my fears whenever

I watched him shy away from the fun, but internally, I was gasping for restorative air and holding back tears.

I braved a consultation with the pediatrician once again, and once again I was told that Luke was perfectly fine. The doctor remained unconcerned that Luke turned away from holiday and party activities that most children anticipate with glee, and he reiterated his opinion that the sudden shaking of Luke's fists, which continued to happen periodically, represented the actions of a very bright, imaginative child who "could be the next Steven Spielberg." No matter how persistently I pointed out that something was wrong with my child, I was dismissed. Mark encouraged me to let it go. He had concluded there was nothing wrong with Luke that firm parenting and time couldn't resolve. Other family members agreed—except for my mother. She alone shared my sadness and bewilderment, and she continued to offer her unconditional support. But even with her encouragement, my nagging self-doubt intensified.

Age four was nonetheless a time of discovery for Luke, and, after watching a television program with us that showcased a violinist, he began insisting he wanted to play the violin. This quest surprised and tickled both Mark and me, and when Luke's interest persisted, we decided there was no harm in trying. It was easy enough to find a rentable child-sized violin, but the search for a violin teacher proved more difficult. Eventually I found a recent immigrant from France who fit the bill, and happily made arrangements for Luke's first lesson with her. That lesson was a brief encounter. As soon as the music teacher began to speak, Luke jumped up and ran out her front door. Making an embarrassed apology, I darted after him, catching him just before he reached the street. And then it dawned on me.

Luke's first nursery school was a cooperative, and on the days when the only mom with a heavy foreign accent was the helper, Luke would invariably run for the door and cling to me as I was leaving. It was a while before I realized it only happened with her, and I found his aversion to her confusing. She was kind and caring. She spoke barely decipherable English, but she smiled a lot, and the other kids seemed to manage just fine. I hadn't initially linked his fear response to her accented speech, but as I watched Luke have such a visceral response to another foreign accent, the dots connected. *But why would a foreign accent create a fear response in Luke?* The questions surrounding his actions and reactions were beginning to mount, and there were no answers in sight.

When Luke continued to talk about violins, however, Mark devised a creative solution. One Saturday, he took Luke to the hardware store, where they purchased a piece of wood about two feet long and a couple of inches thick, some sandpaper, and a can of white paint, which Luke selected. The two of them disappeared into the basement with their purchases and a few pencils in hand. Soon I could hear Luke busily entertaining himself with some toys while Mark went to work with his saw. The next day, the two of them disappeared into the basement again. By Sunday evening, and after many trips up and down the basement stairs, my two favorite people arose from the workbench with Cheshire Cat grins. Luke held something behind his back, and when he saw me, he burst into a big smile. Mark leaned over and whispered something in his ear. Luke nodded and, as he pulled the surprise from behind his back, he raised both arms and said, "Ta-da!" In his hands was an adorable child-sized toy violin, lovingly crafted by father and painted by father and son.

About a month later, Mark and I had plans to celebrate our mid-week wedding anniversary at a local restaurant. When our babysitter phoned and apologetically canceled that afternoon, Luke and I headed to the grocery store, where I selected lamb chops and dinner rolls and Luke helped choose some baby yellow roses. When we returned home, I quickly started dinner and set up a card table in our family room. I covered it with a white cloth and showed Luke how to help set out the utensils and napkins, and then we put the roses in a little vase in the center of the table. I asked if he would like to eat his supper early so he could help serve our food and entertain us with his violin, and he happily agreed to that arrangement.

Hearing the garage door open that evening, Luke ran into the kitchen.

"Dad's here, Mom! Dad's here!"

I wiped the last of the spaghetti sauce from his chin and smoothed down his cowlick, and he ran to greet Mark at the door.

"Dad, come on!" Luke tugged at his dad's hand as he led him into the family room. With a quizzical but pleased expression, Mark removed his coat and set his briefcase on the floor before joining me at the improvised table. I explained the change of plans, and then headed back to the kitchen to plate our food while Mark turned on the stereo. Luke carefully and slowly carried our meals, one at a time, to the table.

"Thank you, kind sir," Mark said with a wink and a smile, and Luke beamed. Mark thought that would likely be the end of Luke's participation, but I indicated he might want to turn around. Luke was standing behind the table with his toy violin nestled under his chin, proudly pretending to glide a bow over imaginary strings, in time with the music playing in the background. I've never before or since enjoyed a meal more than I did that evening. I allowed my fears for Luke's well-being to melt away just a little as the memory of that dinner took hold.

Yet, months later, when it was time to teach Luke to tie his shoelaces, another cause for worry surfaced. Each time we tried over the course of the next several years, Luke's little fingers could not create that bow. Eventually, several years into school, Luke's failure to tie his shoelaces became quite an issue. I worked with Luke; his teachers worked with him, and so did Mark. Occasionally, I would buy shoes without laces, just to give him a break, thinking that the skill would eventually become easy for him. But it never did.

Shoelaces wouldn't seem an obvious trigger to raise concern, but they have come to represent some of my most deeply imprinted memories of the problems Luke faced. Over the years, Luke would, with great deliberation and difficulty, tie a pair of laces on his new shoes once, duplicate that effort to make a double knot, and then struggle every day to stuff his feet into his already-tied shoes, bending the backs of them in the process. He balked at the idea of getting a new pair of shoes when the old ones had outlived their usefulness, no doubt because he didn't want to grapple with new laces. Instead, he clomped around in old shoes tied too loosely and with backs bent beneath his heels, trying desperately to keep his secret.

Luke's internal dialogue on shoes alone must have daily imprinted the thought of "failure" into his psyche. The problem didn't stem from a lack of intelligence. He was a quick learner and asked scientific questions that seemed far beyond his years, yet he couldn't tie his shoelaces. For some reason, his brain-to-hand coordination was out of sync. Questions lingered for me about the connection between Luke's unusual difficulties and the blow to his head, but absent anyone agreeing with me, I learned to keep mostly quiet, realizing the importance of maintaining credibility in all other aspects of Luke's health and development.

Later, we would discover that Luke's attempts at handwriting demonstrated a problem with muscle coordination as well. Throughout his school years, Luke laboriously printed everything he wrote, avoiding cursive writing whenever possible. Forming letters in script overwhelmed him, despite the promise of speedier completion of homework. We bought specially shaped pencils to aid his attempts, to no avail. Teachers suggested he was lazy. I didn't want to encourage or overlook laziness, so I nudged him, but usually backed off when it was obvious he was trying hard, yet not finding success. Luke seemed to me to be anything but lazy. Professionals drawing a conclusion that seemed so at odds with my own observations only deepened my concern and confusion.

My instincts were continually sounding alarms that something was wrong with Luke. But each time I took those concerns to the pediatrician, he dismissed me with a wave of his hand and a laugh. Trying to ground my concerns and balance them with the voice of reason I most trusted, I turned to my mother for advice.

"How is it that one day Luke was a completely adorable, easy child, and the next day he became a stranger and we're left without a road map?"

"I don't know, dear," she would respond, mirroring my worry, "but he has definitely changed."

A Superhero Goes to School

When Luke's fifth birthday arrived in July 1989, I made an appointment to have him tested for kindergarten readiness. The elementary school's only kindergarten teacher liked her boys "to be six," so many families with summer-birthday boys held them back a year to acquiesce to her advice. We decided to have Luke tested anyway, since the pediatrician thought that most of my concerns regarding Luke would fade away once he entered elementary school, assuming all Luke needed was more academic challenge.

During the testing, I sat in a hallway within earshot of the questioning. Asked to use an alphabet chart to identify random letters, Luke retorted with authority, "I'll need your pointer." Apparently that wish was granted, and for the next few minutes, I could hear the tap, tap, tapping on the chart while Luke rapidly identified letter after letter at her command. "You can have this back now," he said, and I could hear her chuckle.

Some basic math questions followed, and then she touched on vocabulary. Luke was a whiz at math for his age and had a sizeable vocabulary, so his answers came quickly, with accuracy and confidence. I sighed and realized I had been holding my breath. It dawned on me that this testing was not only a gauge of Luke's academic readiness for kindergarten, but also an indicator that Luke seemed fine in an all-around sense.

The kindergarten teacher was unhappy that we had decided to enroll Luke in kindergarten at age five, but she couldn't argue with his test results. Academically, Luke was beyond ready to begin school.

When school began that fall, everything went fine—for almost two weeks. Then one morning I received a call from the school secretary, demanding that I come in right away for an unscheduled conference. She wouldn't say why.

Luke had awakened that morning with a stiff and painful leg, having had a booster shot the day before. Suddenly concerned that he had become ill from the injection, I hurried to the school.

As I approached the office, the secretary stood and escorted me to a classroom. The vice principal, the kindergarten teacher, and a language specialist whom I had not previously met were the only people there, and I was directed to sit across from them. Not a word was spoken for what felt like a long time, and the silence was worsened by their three sets of staring eyes. I felt a shudder of intimidation and discomfort. Following a curt introduction to the language specialist, I wondered if Luke needed language therapy of some sort. But why would that require an urgent meeting?

The kindergarten teacher reached down, pulled Luke's backpack from the floor, and handed it to me. In no uncertain terms, she told me that this was his last day of school.

I was dumfounded. "Why?"

The kindergarten teacher spoke first. "Luke thinks he is Batman," she said.

They showed me Luke's drawings of our family (a kindergarten tradition): Mark, Luke, and I were costumed in wonderfully imaginative superhero attire. Luke's drawing of me was captioned "Batmom, heading out to save the world." Mark was decorated with a large "S" on his Superman-blue shirt, and Luke's self-portrait was clearly of Batman himself, hands on his hips and cape flying in the breeze. I found the drawings delightful. "Isn't this what five-year-olds do?" I asked.

I was unprepared for the words I heard next: "We think Luke is psychotic and that he *actually believes* he is Batman."

They had drawn this conclusion because, earlier that morning, Luke had been asked to accompany the language teacher to another room for a standard assessment. He had then jumped into Batman mode and tried to fend her off. He did not attempt to hit or hurt her in any way, but he did try to protect himself, as Batman, from being taken away. Apparently, he thought she was a nurse taking him away for another injection. At first, I thought it was kind of clever from a child's perspective, and recall having a momentary silent laugh as the educators explained their theory. But then it dawned on me that they weren't joking.

So, there we sat. Slack-jawed, I told them I would take their concerns to the pediatrician and also talk with Mark, and get back to them the following day. "No," they insisted collectively. "Luke is going home right now."

Looking back, I wish I had known there were other options to consider, and I wish I had fought them harder. When we arrived home, Luke headed straight to his play corner and busied himself with his building blocks, disinterested in the sudden change of his schedule. I tried to reach Mark at work, but he was in a meeting. Next I phoned and luckily reached the pediatrician, who was as shocked as I had been at the administrators' decision to expel Luke. He said he thought they had made a mistake, but he fell short of advocating for us and told me that keeping Luke home the extra year wouldn't hurt him. *Are you kidding? You told us that what Luke needed was to go to school!* His complacency with the school's actions seemed in direct opposition to his earlier assessment that Luke's difficulties were related to a lack of academic challenge. By this point, however, I was all too familiar with my concerns not making sense to anyone else and realized that pushing for advocacy would only dig a deeper hole.

I decided I needed to keep my anger and frustration at bay. We stood a better chance of helping Luke by holding our ground with this man who in every other way was a good doctor.

I dreaded giving this school news to Mark. With each incident of unexplained and unacceptable behavior from our child, I could feel a wedge being hammered between us, and I hated it.

I awoke the next morning with renewed determination and called the vice principal to ask for an assessment of Luke by the school psychologist, at school expense. "Certainly not," came the response. I insisted. "You made the diagnosis, and it needs to be either professionally supported or refuted." If the school psychologist agreed with their assessment, we needed to enlist their help for Luke; and, if not, the label of "psychotic" needed to be removed from his school file.

Two appointments were grudgingly made for the following week—the first to assess Luke and the second to meet with me. When it was my turn, the school psychologist greeted me with warmth, a kind smile, and more than a minor display of embarrassment. Her first words were to assure me that the school representatives had made a mistake. She told me she had assessed Luke carefully and found that he clearly had a higher than usual anxiety level, but nothing to indicate psychosis.

I've often thought back to that conversation and wondered why I didn't ask for the school's assistance in determining the cause of those high anxiety levels that we all agreed Luke experienced. *Did the nursery school teacher's remarks about abuse still hold sway with me? Had I chickened out subconsciously, not wanting to take the chance that we might again be accused of harming our beloved child?* The rationalization that some children were more anxious about attending school than others was a plausible defense, as was the position that the wait of an extra year would only help Luke. I let it go at that. I felt annoyed that the school representatives had quickly and incorrectly diagnosed Luke, but I was happy that at least the damaging label had been deleted from my son's file. Still, Luke's anxiety and agitation levels *had* caused three professional educators to detect in him something they recognized as abnormal. Psychosis wasn't the cause, but what was?

I decided to take Luke to a private child psychologist for another evaluation during this imposed yearlong delay. After several months of weekly visits, however, she also was unable to figure out Luke's "issues," saying that his manifestations were "highly unusual." She also denied psychosis. I mentioned the accident with the swing, but she concluded that there was no connection to his behavioral difficulties. She suggested that time and maturity would do wonders, and that Luke did not need her help. Goodbye and good luck, basically.

Mark and I considered relocating to give Luke a fresh start for his second try at kindergarten the following September. In the end, though, we decided to stay put, having convinced ourselves that the school would treat Luke fairly, especially since he would then be six, as the kindergarten teacher preferred.

Because of Luke's sudden dismissal from kindergarten, we had to find a prekindergarten option for that year. Fortunately, a little research led to a specialized program in a neighboring town designed just for "summer-five birthday" holdbacks. Thankfully, they had an opening, and Luke jumped into this new routine without any problem and with a measure of enthusiasm. The teachers took his idiosyncrasies in stride, he got along well with the other children, and for the first time in a long while, I thought maturity and time might just return Luke to his former personality.

After school and on weekends, Luke spent much of his time in a small bay window area in our family room that worked beautifully as a play space. Its open shelves allowed him easy access to his toys and games, and he spent hours at a time building with his blocks, never appearing to care or notice if days went by when he didn't see another child.

Not long after Luke's abrupt last day of kindergarten, we discovered in the midst of a downpour that the windows in this area had begun to leak. We hired a contractor who made some cost-saving suggestions. As a result, Luke's well-used play corner would need to be altered. The good news was that an even larger area with toy storage enclosed behind cabinet doors was designed to replace it.

I had told Luke about the scheduled changes, but only when the work had actually begun and he came home from school to find his open shelves and toys no longer there was it apparent that he had not understood. He cried and complained bitterly. I took his hand and walked him over to the new cabinet doors, but Luke turned away. Even when he saw his toys and blocks stacked and ready for play, he continued to cry inconsolably, which struck me as out of proportion to the situation.

This went on for weeks, and then months—far too long to categorize as normal, at least by my opinion. And Luke's fixation and inability to adapt to this small modification in his environment raised another red flag: *what does obsession to this degree mean?* Mark and I both grew increasingly frustrated with Luke's escalating behavioral malfunctioning.

I tried everything I could think of to redirect Luke's attention from his familiar corner. Ignoring his negative behavior had no impact; neither did associating the new play area with fun activities. Lacking any other parental insights or knowledge, more often than not I left Luke to cry it out on his own, assuming that ignoring his outbursts would eventually effect change. Over the months, Luke's hysteria calmed somewhat, but he remained upset by that play corner change for years, and he reminded me about it whenever it crossed his mind. Luke's tenacious fixations were anything but charming, and I tried my best to not take his anger personally.

I sought help from extended family members. I longed for someone, anyone, to believe me and to recognize that Luke needed more help than we were able to provide. Instead, they told me I should learn how to be a more effective parent, and that because Luke had behavioral difficulties, I was obviously not doing my stay-at-home job correctly.

By this point, I was enervated from trying to neutralize Luke's outbursts. My lack of confidence deepened. To try to solve the problem,

I built quite a collection of child-rearing books, read everything I could get my hands on, and tried many of the suggestions, but to no avail. There were some tricks I hadn't thought of, but they produced no lasting changes in Luke's behavior. Much of the material was based on common sense, which helped to reinforce what we were already doing. Other books espoused techniques we opposed, like spanking, so they were of no use.

I continued to watch other parents with their children, which added to my confusion. My parenting style seemed consistent with theirs. It utilized distracting and redirecting tactics, focused on positives, ignored negative behaviors as much as possible, and included a lot of warmth and hugs as integral ingredients. I tried to be consistent and could be firm when the situation called for it, just like every successful parent I had studied. *Why were my efforts falling so short of adequate?*

When Luke turned six, I set out to put my instinctive unease to rest once and for all. I saved household money and made an appointment with a young pediatric neurologist who had just opened a practice in our area. I never told Mark or the pediatrician that I was taking Luke for another assessment because I knew they would discourage it and tell me I was reacting to a baseless fear. But I remained convinced that the changes in my son were a direct result of the accident with the swing three years earlier. If I was right, surely a pediatric neurologist would uncover the connection.

Luke and I arrived a few minutes early for the appointment, but had a forty-five minute wait to see the doctor. By the time we were finally called in, Luke's agitation level had escalated, and he was difficult to console or contain. The young doctor managed to get Luke to do a few basic exercises, like touching his fingers to his nose and walking a straight line. He looked at Luke's spine and checked his reflexes. Everything he tested was normal, but I wanted him to test behavioral responses instead of, or at least in addition to, reflexes. I had explained the reason for our visit, but to my dismay, the physician dismissed my concerns as unrelated to the blow to Luke's head. He did, however, tell me that he saw Luke as a "behavioral problem" and "impulsive." As Luke darted around the examining room and was obviously difficult to corral, the doctor led us to the door.

His parting words are ones I will never forget. He leaned against the door, looked me in the eyes, and said, "You just need to be a better mother."

My knees weakened. I thought I might be sick. What I had anticipated as a chance for hope instead closed in and smothered me. *If this professional, trained in the workings of a child's brain, denied any connection between the blow to Luke's head and his sudden but lasting behavioral changes, then what was causing them?*

For the next several days, I alternated between defensive anger at the doctor and everyone else who didn't believe me, and the fear that they might be correct. I felt strangely and frustratingly out of sync with the very people I needed in my corner.

I had counted on Luke's unexpected delay in entering kindergarten to work out in the end, and on him maturing out of his difficulties. But that wasn't what happened. On the contrary, his "new" personality was becoming only more entrenched and challenging. He would often hyperfocus, and his inability to adapt, adjust, and "let go" worsened. His hyperactivity manifested not so much in physical movement as in mental agitation, which was palpable and disturbing to watch. His eyes often took on a wild expression, matching behavior that was difficult to contain. He was a child for whom few redirectional attempts were effective. Feeding Luke protein at the first sign of a meltdown and allowing extra time to rest were the only things I found that provided any hint of help.

Yet the pediatrician stuck to his belief that Luke's heightened activity was a manifestation of his significant intelligence combined with a powerful imagination. I tried hard to be consoled by those words, but they didn't ring true for me. Something was wrong with my son and time was being wasted in my search to uncover it and find help for him.

In spite of Luke's change of personality following the accident with the swing, he remained the joy of my life. I worried constantly about his "differences" relative to other children, but I held onto hope that he would level off. My initial sense of panic at the moment of impact had been transformed into a simmering unease that bubbled over when specific problems arose. Through it all, Luke maintained a sweetness that often overrode his high levels of agitation and anxiety. It is difficult to know if my love for Luke was even greater than it might have been if he had not had problems; I only know that I loved him beyond measure and admired his determination to overcome whatever those undefined problems were.

Of all my cherished memories of Luke, one that is particularly vivid is how he learned to settle into bedtime. The intense anxiety that he displayed each evening, beginning immediately after the accident, eventually morphed into a stoic acceptance of the inevitability of being left alone to find sleep, but not without heavy tugs to my heartstrings.

Mark and I had continued to read a story to Luke every night. My turn usually followed Mark's, and when I was finished, I would kiss Luke on the forehead, tell him I loved him, and tuck him in. Although he remained visibly distressed, a bittersweet pattern emerged over time. Night after night, Luke would look up at me with an expression of innocence mixed with agitation. He would pat his book, raise his eyebrows, and offer the cutest wry smile, as if to say, "Just one more chapter, Mom, please?" "Tomorrow is another day," I would tell him as I kissed his head again. Without exception, he would reach up and throw his arms around my neck in a tight hug before giving in to the inevitable. Looking back at this time in Luke's life, I am touched by his ability to manage his internal anxiety with humor and grace, and am saddened to the core that he had to.

Academically, Luke did fine in his second try at kindergarten, and that encouraging trend continued for the next four or five years of schooling. Socially, however, he faced many challenges, which his teachers pronounced a matter of immaturity, and which his classmates' parents viewed as reasons to avoid him. Although Luke's natural sweetness prevailed most of the time, it was comingled with perceptible agitation that always seemed to lie just below the surface, ready to manifest in action at any moment. Although Luke was not a behavioral handful in school, I'm guessing that his unsettled demeanor was reason enough for other parents to want their kids to look past Luke to other children for playmates. That realization was heartbreaking, both in the moment and over time. It was also beyond frustrating because, as a mother, I wondered if I might not have taken the same approach if the situation had been reversed. I would like to think not, but, lacking the insights that have naturally fallen into place for me in dealing with Luke's difficulties, the truth is I likely would not have understood any more than those parents did.

At the close of his second first day of kindergarten, I stood outside the school behind a group of other kindergarten parents. They were busy exchanging phone numbers and setting up playdates for their kids, and they did not see me. I overheard one of the moms admonishing the others to not let their children play with Luke. I couldn't see her facial expression, just the back of her head shaking back and forth as the others laughed. We lived in a small town, and parents sized up their children's potential friends quickly. I have no way of knowing how this mother had formed her premature judgment about Luke, but my guess is his fist-shaking episodes had become common fodder for gossip during those prekindergarten years.

It didn't take long for the boys to be labeled as either popular or unpopular—a practice led mostly by the parents. A distinct separation between the two groups formed. Luke, unsurprisingly, fell into the unpopular category, and my attempts to arrange playdates for him with any of the "popular" boys were futile. Parents from Luke's group were more laid-back, as were their sons, and were usually accommodating and reciprocating in setting up time for our boys to play together. Luke, however, often remained disinterested. He seemed content to come home after school, complete his one or two pages of homework, and then retreat to his new play corner (which he had finally come to accept, but never to like) to quietly build with his blocks for hours on end.

Luke played soccer in the fall of his first-grade year along with the rest of his classmates, despite not yet understanding the basic concepts of the game. The kids looked cute in their uniform tee shirts, running up and down the field and chasing the mostly elusive ball. Luke ran gleefully beside them—with one huge difference. While the other kids ran in a pack and tried to get to the ball, Luke just ran up and down the field— apparently having no idea there even was a ball, and seemingly unaware there were teammates.

Luke's obliviousness on the soccer field was repeated on the baseball diamond that spring. Again, Luke appeared lost in the process of learning the sport and had difficulty hitting, throwing, and catching the ball. During one game, he managed to get to first base. Waiting for something else to happen, he became distracted, knelt down, and began building a castle in the dirt. His focus was on his construction project, so much so that he never realized a teammate had gotten a hit and that he should advance to the next base. Despite cries from his teammates and coaches to "Run, Luke, run," he never looked up from his castle.

While many children that age can be unfocused in the art of learning a sport, the level of Luke's disconnect from his surroundings was well beyond what seemed normal to Mark and me. It was also beyond what appeared normal to the other kids and their parents, and they were quick to point that out.

Although he was willing to attend practices and games for various sports, Luke remained otherwise satisfied to stay in his play corner at home for hours at a time. I grew anxious about his social disinterest; he seemed content to be alone at an age when other children were forming friendships and learning how to maneuver through the complexities of socialization. Struggling to be the better mother that my family and Luke's doctors expected, I secretly continued to search for clues to the source of his difficulties. But I didn't know where to look, and trips to the library to research possibilities left me even more frustrated when I found no answers.

Luke continued to want to play recreational soccer and baseball in spite of his conspicuous disengagement from the purpose of the games and from the teamwork inherent in them. In third grade, the parent coaches began to teach the children basketball. Once again, Luke, an enthusiastic participant, ran up and down the court but failed to connect with the object of the game and with the concept of passing the ball back and forth. As I watched him fail in his attempts to learn week after week, my heart broke for him. I prayed that until his abilities caught up, he would remain unaware that his participation in the game was not in the same league as his teammates', and that he would never hear their ugly comments about him.

It was so easy to conclude that my son was a sensitive and dreamy child, unadept at sports. I could not see that this was yet another piece of a puzzle, the full picture of which would show an injured brain. Luke would continue to provide clues over the next ten or so years, some subtle and some quite obvious.

If only we had known what to look for . . .

The Color of His Nines

One day, as eight-year-old Luke sat next to me in the car, he broke the easy quiet of the ride with a question: "Mom, what color are your nines?"

Startled, I replied to his question with one of my own. "I'm not sure, Luke. What do you mean?"

"You know, Mom, when you think of a number, what color is it?"

I thought for a moment, and then hesitated before replying, "I'm still not sure what you mean. Can you describe it for me?"

"Well, my nines are blue, and my fours are green. You know, Mom, how every number is a different color."

"Oh, that must be fun!" I replied, trying to hold at bay a gnawing sense of worry.

Several weeks later, Luke asked the question again, and again I did not know how to respond. But he was so insistent that, as soon as he had gone to school the next day, I telephoned the pediatrician for his advice.

As I might have expected, the pediatrician was unconcerned about Luke visualizing numbers in separate, distinct colors. "I keep telling you," he said, "Luke will be the next Steven Spielberg. Let it go!" And so I did.

With no one to relate to his visions of color, Luke let it go as well. He had likely hoped I would have a quick and easy explanation for him, and that I would tell him I knew just what he meant. But I could not, and he never mentioned it to me again. I've often wondered what he internalized about experiencing those colors that no one else saw.

The preadolescent years, which sparked more and more social

awareness among his peers, continued to see Luke left in the dark, and his maturation lag became more evident with the passage of time. Having been labeled an unpopular kid since kindergarten, he had a lot of territory to cover to gain acceptance, but thankfully, in the early grades at least, he stayed sweetly oblivious to the social exclusions.

Until fourth grade, Luke also remained tuned out to the fads that enticed his classmates. But that year, he caught on with enthusiasm, although usually during a given fad's waning phase. Midway through the school year, "milk caps"—small, flat cardboard discs decorated with pictures—became instant must-haves among the kids. I had noticed the kids playing games and wearing plastic tubes that held the milk caps hanging by strings around their necks, but several weeks went by before Luke took notice. Once he did, however, he jumped into the activity wholeheartedly.

One day after school, he ran to his room and retrieved his piggy bank. Then he ran back down the hallway and asked if I would take him to the variety store, right away! There was urgency in his voice. I was thrilled with this sudden interest in a social activity, and we got in the car and set out. Luke was bouncier than usual during the short ride, and at the store he painstakingly made his milk cap selection. Thereafter, week after week, he wore the green plastic tube he'd selected, filled with his disc treasures, displaying more excitement about those toys than I'd seen him show for anything in years. For the first time in a long time, his exuberance overrode my confusion and fears for his future.

That fad came and went quickly through the school, but not for Luke. He clung to those discs long after his classmates had replaced them with the next passing fancy. He took them off only to shower and sleep at night (at our insistence), but during the day they hung around his neck constantly. The other children mocked him, as milk caps had become yesterday's news, yet Luke seemed unaware of their derision. Trying to spare him, we encouraged him to leave the green tube at home when he went to school, but he remained innocently oblivious, and his interest held on for weeks.

Lagging social awareness was just one aspect of Luke's difficulties. I was much more concerned about his basic cluelessness in navigating the world around him. This was not a child who could be trusted to look both ways before crossing a street, or who would be able to find his way home from several blocks away. By age ten, Luke hadn't yet begun to engage with his surroundings. Common sense told me that this connection was a gradual process for any child, but I kept waiting for that *click* of emerging recognition to appear on his face or in his actions—recognition of where he was relative to the world around him. It wasn't happening, not even remotely.

His innocence presented greater challenges with every passing year. Instead of trusting that Luke would be okay when his class took an all-day field trip, I worried that he might wander off if he wasn't carefully watched. As opportunities arose for Luke to experience life at distances farther and farther from home, I never knew how far to stretch my concerns to allow him those normal freedoms. I watched as other kids his age proved themselves capable of handling age-appropriate freedom and responsibility, and it was painful to admit to myself that Luke was not even close to achieving those milestones. Luke was the proverbial babe in the woods, and the constant efforts I made to help him connect the dots and bring him up to speed were showing few, if any, results.

Later that year, Luke was invited to spend an evening with a classmate and his parents at an amusement park several hours from home. This child was as close to a friend as my son would have in elementary school, and neither he nor Luke seemed to care about not being at the center of the social scene at school. This night away from home could be a fun experience for a child of ten, but Luke was ten in numerical age only. Making the decision more difficult was our observation that his friend's parents embraced a laissez-faire child-rearing style. Mark and I liked them very much, but realized that their approach would likely be to arrive at this huge park, frequented at night mostly by older teens and adults, and just let the kids go off to have fun without checking on them periodically. For another child, that approach might be harmless. But Luke could and would wander away without realizing it and be easy prey for bullying or worse by the older crowd. If he became separated from his friend, he most likely would not find his way back to the family.

The decision itself was straightforward; neither Mark nor I leaned in the direction of saying yes. We did offer to go along and spend the evening with his friend's parents, but they were celebrating an anniversary and had planned this as a "date night." In the end, there was nothing to do but decline the invitation, wishing it could be different.

Luke held onto intense disappointment about this perceived missed opportunity for years. He periodically brought it up well into his teens, and each time he did, his anger intensified. Although we never doubted the soundness of our decision, we found his inability to let go of his disappointment, even years later, troubling.

Otherwise, at ten, Luke still loved to hug and to laugh, and he seemed unaware of the slights by teachers, classmates, and their parents that were painfully obvious to me. As a classroom mom, I observed both the occasional rolling of the teachers' eyes when Luke would appear distracted, and the way the popular crowd and their parents avoided social interaction with him. But, mostly, Luke was sweet and loveable, intelligent but clueless and undeterred, and his enthusiasm could be a joy to behold.

As a preteen, Luke began to ask what I thought were insightful academic questions, often about the laws of physics. Whenever Luke stumped me with his questions, he would turn to his dad and, from that, a deepening father-son bond emerged. The two of them would hash through scientific topics, and I loved the sight of them huddled together. And, although Luke's reading skills were for some unknown reason not keeping pace, he handled without obvious difficulty the academic requirements of the elementary school years. It was easy enough at this point to give in to my hopes and dreams for Luke by assigning his lagging reading and social skills and unawareness of his surroundings to the simplicity of delayed maturity. When I was honest with myself, I knew some other cause lurked more deeply. Yet I fell prey to believing what I wanted to believe and rationalized that, if his pediatrician and teachers weren't uncovering anything more serious, maybe there really was nothing to worry about. I wanted so badly to believe that.

Luke seemed to enjoy school, and he reveled in his academic successes during those early years. To help encourage his interest in education, we took a road trip to a small historical town nearby. Dinner that evening included historic food options, with entertainment and service by people dressed in period costume. The tables were crafted from heavy, rough-hewn wood topped with tall, lit candles, which were the room's only source of illumination. As I passed a saltshaker to Mark, my arm knocked one of the candles over. Mark quickly extinguished the small flame, and as the moment of excitement passed, Luke, with eyes a little wider than normal and the corners of his mouth turned up into a small smile, looked across at me. "I thought for a moment you were going to have to stop, drop, and roll!" Here was a socially lagging child making a factual, learned statement with a touch of laid-back humor, while sounding a bit like a precious old sage.

As we toured historic sites that weekend, I chose to walk slightly behind my two favorite men as they stopped at every informative marker. Luke watched as his dad read each plaque, and he took the same stance as his father, with his hands clasped similarly behind his back. He looked seriously at the markers, and began moving his lips, pretending to read every word that Mark read. He obviously idolized Mark. I wished I could bottle that weekend and apply it every time worry about Luke surfaced.

Mark had been an avid Boy Scout, and he easily accepted the role of scoutmaster when the boys in Luke's school formed a troop. Interest in scouting waned quickly for most of his classmates, but there were kids a year older than Luke who actively participated, so with Mark's encouragement, Luke decided to stay the course. For several weeks that fall, father and son disappeared each evening into the basement to work on their pinewood derby car. Although their car didn't win, the fun of trying enticed Luke to remain a scout, even though by fourth grade he was the only one in his class to still wear the uniform to school one day each week.

Luke's first weekend camping adventure occurred that winter, and ten-year-old Luke, with some help from Mark, headed off to the campsite with another scout leader and the older scouts. The site was only about ten miles from home, which eased my worry. The fact that someone other than Mark was assigned to oversee the overnight segment was, we originally thought, a good thing. Luke needed an infusion of self-reliance and camaraderie. But I was so concerned about his tenacious cluelessness about the world around him that at 6:00 o'clock the following morning, in the midst of a heavy and cold February downpour, I asked Mark to go and check on Luke. As one of the best gifts he would ever give me, Mark left his newspaper and steaming cup of coffee and drove to the sodden campsite while I breathed a sigh of relief. Luke had survived the experience just fine, and thankfully never realized his dad was doing anything but participating in his role as scoutmaster.

As Luke grew older, the sense that he was like a child lost in the woods grew ever stronger in me. I couldn't put my finger on why; Luke was certainly not helpless. He could dress himself and take care of his basic needs without assistance. Yet there was something palpably "different" about him: he remained disengaged.

Luke's teachers continued to laud his innate academic abilities, and his IQ scores reinforced their observations. *Was Luke just slow to mature, as some of them suggested? Was he lazy and manipulative, as others said he was?* To me, nothing about him seemed lazy; he was just the opposite, in fact. Luke wanted to succeed; that much was obvious to me. He began every project with enthusiasm, only to weary and give up as his undefined difficulties became insurmountable. I had watched him do exactly that time and time again. And when he failed, his sweet face showed signs that he blamed himself, worsening his chances at future success.

Mark and I were happy that Luke had maintained his interest in playing recreational team sports throughout his first four or five years of school, but after a few years of observing his continued disconnect in soccer, baseball, and then basketball, I finally took my concerns to the pediatrician. Accustomed by now to the doctor's dismissals, I steeled myself to be ignored again. This time, to my surprise and relief, he gave consideration to Luke's sporting difficulties and said that Luke might be more successful at individual rather than team sports. He suggested tennis and golf.

We accepted his advice, and I thanked Mark for providing for our family well enough that we could offer that opportunity to Luke. Tennis came first. Luke took to it better than we thought he might. It was a revelation to watch his ability to follow the rules of that game, and also to find a level of success with it. While never a prodigy, he managed to hold his own in some local competitions, resulting in a shy smile that lingered on his face during the drive home.

With tennis a success, we eventually added golf. Mark already played, so I decided to learn along with Luke, thinking ahead to family outings and vacations that might center on the sport. Luke was by then about twelve years old, and he exhibited a strong natural talent for this new game. His difficulties with it were emotional rather than physical, and he occasionally refused to move on when he hit a bad shot. Although he understood that other players were waiting behind him, he was obsessive—and adamant—about trying again and again until he hit the ball correctly. At first, we thought his behavior was a case of preteen belligerence, and we clamped down to stop it quickly.

But Luke only held tightly to his demand to stay put. Whenever we went out on the course, I could feel my stomach muscles tighten in anticipation of the argument that could easily ensue. Luke's behavior was infuriating. It was also confusing. Although golf is known to bring out the worst in some people, these weren't simply bad moments for Luke. Days afterward, he remained agitated about not having been able to redo his bad shots, despite being reminded of the people behind him waiting to play. His foul mood held on, far outlasting an everyday bratty tantrum.

Mark and I didn't let up on him. In order to get back on the course, Luke had to apologize and let go of his anger. When he finally did, we would take him golfing again. Good behavior, good fun. The concept was simple enough and sometimes it seemed to work, but other times, often when we least expected it, Luke's discontent would be suddenly triggered without a clear cause. We never knew what any given day would bring in terms of Luke's impulsivity and outbursts.

We were saddened to add golf to the list of situations in which Luke failed to make the connection between his actions and their consequences. Still, I clung to hope that his enjoyment of both tennis and golf might provide the incentive he needed to learn to conform to the rules of the games. If he matured into an understanding of those "actions to consequences" connections, then he might also begin to connect those dots to life in general. He had to; something had to happen soon to help pull Luke out of this deepening mire of failure.

Growing Into Injury

Fifth grade incorporated some significant educational shifts, including test questions requiring in-depth answers. And fifth grade was when Luke's cognitive difficulties emerged to show themselves clearly.

Luke had managed well in previous grades when he was able to fill in the blanks with one-word answers, select from multiple choices, or circle "True" or "False." Earlier-grade teachers had been grooming the students to take on more responsibility with group activities, lessons on how to conduct research, and class discussions. But conferences with Luke's teachers highlighted his disengagement from group participation and his inability to grasp research skills. One teacher summarized it as "stubborn disinterest in learning new concepts." I had no concrete evidence beyond maternal observation, but I tried to persuade her that Luke did want to succeed, and that he took pride in his successes. I suggested that his failure to keep pace might point to a developmental problem. She lowered her face and looked at me over the top of her glasses for a long moment. Then she said, "Luke is not trying, and that is what you need to take away from this meeting."

Because the layering of education is a gradual, cumulative process, it is logical to assume that any student who misses a concept here and a concept there will eventually be unable to keep pace. Logic would again predict that the earlier the missing gaps are recognized and remediated, the better the chances for the student to reach his or her potential. Luke was beginning to fit into the "missed concepts" category, and although some of his educational miscues were being recognized, I felt the school was not addressing them. Instead of viewing Luke's accumulating lapses as signs of a larger problem, they chose to blame him, despite his nearly straight-A record up to this point. Several of his teachers still referred to him as "lazy" and assumed he only had to try harder.

By the fifth grade, reading assignments were no longer short books with simple words, and reports began to require multiple steps for completion. Like every other advancing student, Luke now needed to follow complex instructions, but he was noticeably slower to catch on, at least according to reports from teachers and from Mark's and my observations at home. *Did he just need a little extra push and a little extra time before multistep assignments would begin to make sense?* We encouraged Luke's efforts at home and often sat nearby as he tackled homework, but unfortunately, he grew only more and more tentative and uneasy as his educational responsibilities increased. As the school year progressed and he realized that for the first time he wasn't keeping up with his classmates, Luke's enthusiasm for school began to wane, and a visible disquietude took its place.

One day in early spring, I was assigned to visit Luke's classroom to help the teacher with a project. I wasn't there long when she said to the children, "Class, shall we tell Luke's mom what Luke does every day? There he goes again, class, *tap, tap, tap* with his pencil!" I walked up to her, glared into her eyes, and spoke softly so the children wouldn't hear: "Please do not ever say that again." She looked at me quizzically, as though my request made no sense to her. I left the classroom that day insecure about Luke's emotional safety there, yet without a concrete way to stop it from happening again. I kept as close an eye as possible on the situation for the few remaining months of the school year, counting on the administrators to follow up on my complaint and keep their eyes on Luke's emotional well-being, but I remained concerned.

At about this same time, Mark and I began to notice that when Luke had to write something, he never expanded on thoughts in any detail or depth. His ability to think and process information orally—by talking—

43

was better, but only slightly. It was frustratingly difficult to try to extract information from Luke in any detail. Whether it was a thank-you note for a birthday gift, or the answer to a homework question asking *why* or *how*, the end result was word-poor.

As expanded answers were increasingly required on tests, Luke did not grow into the task, but only continued this word-deficient pattern. One- or two-word responses eventually grew into one or two sentences, but his teachers wanted more, understandably. No matter how hard we tried, or how we changed tactics to help Luke put his thoughts and knowledge into words, that skill eluded him. It was frustrating mostly because we couldn't determine what was holding him back, and had no idea how to find out. He was, according to both standardized IQ measurements and personal observation, a bright child. He manifested his grasp of a subject best through verbal communication, however, which made traditional schooling a difficult match for him.

Middle school officially began that fall with Luke's entry into sixth grade, but since this was a K-8 school, there was really nothing "official" about it. The middle-schoolers did change classrooms for their various subjects instead of having the same teacher all day, and we anticipated this conversion to budding autonomy as a healthy shift for Luke. Getting up and walking to a different classroom every forty minutes or so might energize him and light a fire of intellectual curiosity.

I noticed a slight lifting of the academic unease that had begun the previous year. *Could the pediatrician be correct after all that nothing was wrong with Luke except the need to allow his innate intellect room to grow? Had Luke managed to remediate those small but obvious gaps in his educational foundation?* Fighting against intuition to the contrary, I began to allow optimism some space to take hold.

My reprieve from worry did not last long; in fact, the pediatrician's theory that intellectual challenge was all Luke needed basically imploded. By the end of the first sixth-grade marking period, Luke's various teachers made it clear that Luke was missing deadlines in every subject, failing to complete assignments altogether, and consistently forgetting to arrive to class prepared with the correct book, notebooks, and pen. Luke listened well in the classroom, however, so his test results were adequate to keep his grades at a passing level and, in many cases, well above. This was our first experience having more than one teacher for Luke in the same school year, and Mark and I weren't prepared for those multiple reports that our son was an unfocused, unprepared, slacking student. We knew that middle school observations can help to identify areas of study or behavior that need more attention, and that bringing the parents on board and recruiting their assistance can benefit the child in catching up. For Mark and me, however, these were stunning observations, and we were beyond our abilities to know how to help him.

During Luke's early elementary school years, conferences with his classroom teachers generally included the message that, in spite of trying and making some headway, he continued to lag socially. Even the teacher conferences that had alluded to a "lazy" tendency to avoid learning new skills hadn't prepared us for these multiple reports of Luke not doing well in school.

Mark and I tried to increase Luke's responsibilities at home, hoping that would help. Unfortunately, that just dug a deeper hole for Luke, since he was still woefully lacking in his ability to make connections between actions and consequences. Raising the bar for him only increased that gap, and we watched as Luke became sullen and emotionally withdrawn as the year progressed.

"Noises in My Head"

As a young teen, Luke approached me hesitantly one morning and said, "Can I ask you something, Mom?" Having become uncomfortably accustomed to his withdrawn demeanor and aversion to expanded conversation, I aimed for nonchalance, hoping he wouldn't back away. "Sure, Luke."

"There are noises in my head," he began. "It's like there are five televisions going at once, and I can't turn them off. Do you know how?"

This was certainly not what I had expected or hoped to hear, and his words felt like a punch to the gut. Trying to appear calm, and not knowing what to say, I began with some questions. Were the noises there when he tried to go to sleep? Did they sound like people talking, or were they more like banging, clanging sounds?

"I don't know, Mom. There's so much noise and it won't stop."

Tension built inside me, but I tried hard to mask my fears. It isn't every day that your child enlists your help for noises he hears in his head that can't be quieted.

I hugged him and thanked him for letting me know, then stooped slightly to eye level and looked at him intently. "I promise I will do all I can to learn what is causing this so those noises stop," I said. He gave that sweet smile I so loved.

And while Luke was in school that day, I once again turned to the pediatrician for help. Surely, this would get his attention.

"I keep telling you Luke will be the next Steven Spielberg," came the immediate reply, with a slight hint of annoyance in his voice. "Luke is just highly imaginative and highly intelligent. This is nothing to worry about." After I made several attempts to challenge that line of thinking, the conversation ended, and once again I felt as though I had been kindly scolded for asking a stupid question and taking time away from the doctor's more important matters, like treating children who were actually sick. And, because this physician had been so on-target over the years with his diagnoses of Luke's ear infections and flu and viruses, I felt an added sense of humiliation for continuing to harp on a subject that obviously had no validity in his eyes.

By this point, I had learned the art of acquiescing. My multiple attempts over the years to convince medical and educational professionals that Luke's playground accident had significantly altered his behavior and personality had been universally ignored. The pediatrician, a child psychologist, a pediatric neurologist, and Luke's teachers had all tossed my concerns into the "overinvolved mother" basket and, lacking their professional credentials, I had fallen prey to their pronouncements, losing a considerable amount of self-assurance in the process.

Not knowing where else to turn, I next tried to locate any reference to "noises in the head" in the parenting library I had amassed, but found nothing. I also asked coworkers at the church where I worked part-time, and was given a lead to a psychologist whose own child had encountered years of classroom difficulties. Because Luke continued to be the target of bullying behavior from some of his classmates and their parents, and even from some teachers, I told myself that taking him to see a psychologist at this point was likely a good idea anyway. Luke didn't seem to mind the appointments, and I assumed he was comfortable talking about his difficulties, knowing that the counselor's own son had also had a hard time in school. The psychologist was unfortunately not able to determine a cause for the "noises" Luke described, however, and he, too, minimized their importance.

"Luke is internally very anxious," he told me, adding, "yet I can't seem to put my finger on why." I had heard that phrase before, certainly. *What, exactly, did "can't seem to put my finger on it" mean? Was it something he had never encountered before, or was it too minor to be a causative factor?* He went on to explain that Luke could seem very calm one moment, but then quickly show signs of agitation by reacting strongly to a seemingly neutral subject without being able to verbalize what was bothering him. Luke's displays of agitation were all too familiar to me; I had seen them too many times since his head had been struck by the swing to not recognize the psychologist's description. Agitation in Luke at this age manifested as a suddenly discomforted facial expression, a rapid flicking of his foot, and an inability to sit still.

The psychologist suggested Luke would likely outgrow this, and that the noises he alluded to were perhaps a few manifestations of puberty that a sensitive, imaginative boy had found a creative way to describe. *Likely. Perhaps.* These words did not instill confidence that this psychologist had a grip on the source of Luke's difficulties.

So, in spite of Luke's recent transition from an adorable and talkative yet agitated boy to a quiet, agitated adolescent who kept to himself and had begun to flounder academically, I challenged myself to accept this assessment at face value. I had never been a boy; I had never experienced adolescence from the male perspective, and I had to trust that this was all normal for my son. Besides, Mark thought Luke's withdrawal from us was completely age-appropriate.

"But did you ever hear noises in your head?" I asked him.

"Not that I can remember, but who knows? It's likely nothing."

I wanted desperately to believe that, so eventually I let it go. Although the worry refused to ease completely, I rationalized most of it away by telling myself that since Luke had only mentioned the "noises" a few times, they were likely nothing to worry about.

A Teenager Emerges

With the arrival of his teen years, Luke became increasingly distant and uncommunicative. He remained hidden away in his room after school, and it was difficult to draw him out and engage him in after-school and summer activities. Computers were not the magnets that they are today, but Luke became engrossed in video games, so much so that he needed redirection to keep from spending hour after hour in front of the screen. He also developed an intense interest in heavy metal music that made me uncomfortable, mostly because of its often angry and misogynistic lyrics.

Whether connected to the games and music or not, Luke's displays of disrespect toward me rose to an intolerable level, and I doubled my efforts to neutralize the tendency. I imposed natural consequences, hoping to promote enjoyment of the rewards that came with showing respect. Consequences still did not seem to impact Luke, and although I kept expecting that as he got older they would, that didn't happen. Instead, he faced homework and chores with increasing stubbornness and defiance, never comprehending that his cooperation would result in better grades, fewer calls from teachers, and time to play afterward. Nothing I tried seemed to work in the face of Luke's inertia. He appeared tired and inactive all the time. I waffled between being angry with him and questioning myself as my efforts failed.

The only breaks in his inertia involved sports. His interest in golf and tennis increased over time, and Mark and I delighted in the possibility that he would learn some valuable life lessons from participating. With indoor tennis available year-round, we arranged for weekly lessons with a young coach who took Luke's personality quirks in stride. Under his tutelage, Luke entered a few tournaments that required travel to other areas of the state. While he never excelled, he did seem to gain a bit of self-confidence with each opportunity. The tournaments also provided chances for us to be together as a family, which was both a joy and a source of anxiety, since Luke's mood had begun to darken. I chalked it up to adolescent hormones, and hoped they would even out quickly and that his tendency to withdraw from us would reverse.

Tennis wasn't a popular sport among his classmates, but in the spring of Luke's sixth-grade year, the gym coach decided to teach the kids to play on a couple of old town-owned courts behind the school. While most of the students had difficulty at first just getting the ball over the net, Luke was able to slam serves across and show a degree of finesse on the court. He came home from school that day wearing his wry little grin, proud to share with us his personal coup.

Luke also continued to play team sports at the recreational level, and his determination to persevere despite obvious failures provided an element of hope that he would soon outgrow his difficult adolescence. In the winter of his seventh-grade year, he was assigned to a basketball team that consisted mostly of athletic eighth-graders who also played on competitive traveling teams. The parent coach was both astute and kind, and he recognized in Luke a desire to fit in. During practice sessions, he instructed the more advanced players to pass the ball to Luke, so over the course of the season, Luke's ball-handling abilities improved, as did his confidence. Luke did not become a great player, but he was finally included as "one of the guys." The team went on to have a championship year, and Luke enjoyed the fruits of their success alongside them. Watching him make some baskets and pass the ball back and forth was joyful for Mark and me, but the best part was the sense of confidence and belonging Luke experienced as part of this team. For him, this level of social acceptance was a rarity.

Unfortunately, a dismal experience on a recreational baseball team in the spring of Luke's eighth-grade year erased the confidence he had gained in basketball. That parent coach was deadly serious about training a winning team, and he had little patience for mistakes. Luke was a bottom-rung addendum to his roster of mostly travel-team boys. During one game, Luke got to first base on a walk, but then was tagged out for not getting back to base in time. His teammates jumped out of their seats and began to hit the wire fence with their fists and mitts, shouting "You idiot, Luke!" And then, very loudly, the coach too called Luke an idiot. I was astounded. Every fiber in me wanted to jump down from the stands and ask that parent coach what kind of an idiot *he* was for disrespecting my son. I remember rocking back and forth on the bleacher seat, holding back tears.

Several innings later, one of the other players, talented and well respected, was also called out at first base, exactly the way Luke had been. But this time the bench was quiet. Suddenly I heard Luke's voice call out through the silence, "Good try!" *How could this sweet boy, still reeling from the insults hurled at him just thirty minutes earlier, continue to be so kind?* Luke, having borne the brunt of many an insult, had apparently learned empathy for others in the process, and that thrilled my mother-heart.

Mark was away on a business trip, so I phoned the coach that evening to express my outrage. He told me unapologetically that his job was to make sure his team won, adding that he had no patience for a kid who couldn't "cut it." It was an obvious waste of my time and energy to continue the conversation. I remember feeling depleted and exhausted for Luke that night, trying to look happy while letting him know how proud I was that he had encouraged his teammate. And in return, Luke displayed one of his priceless smiles before retreating into his room, shoulders slumped.

By seventh and eighth grade, Luke's academic and social struggles became entrenched, and he evolved into a master of deflection. The nagging internal voice that told me all was not right with the world grew ever louder. I cannot begin to imagine the scope of Luke's own internal dialogue. But one thing was clear: he was working very hard to hide his academic inefficacies and to divert attention from them by making poor behavioral choices. The more defensive and deflective Luke became, the more evident his self-loathing. *But why? And where would this lead if the cause for it was not soon uncovered?*

We didn't realized it at the time, but this was a turn in the road for Luke, after which he would never again find a safe haven.

Reading, Writing, 'Rithmatic

Middle school attached deadlines to assignments that involved higher-level chapter books, so Mark and I dedicated time in the evenings to reading with Luke. One night I noticed that, although Luke seemed focused on reading his book, long periods of time would elapse before he turned a page. Catching Mark's eye, I nodded toward the kitchen where, out of earshot of Luke, I shared my observations. Within minutes, Mark returned to the kitchen ashen-faced. "I don't think Luke can read," he said, quickly adding, "but I know he can. I've heard him read aloud any number of times. What's going on?"

We decided to request a reading assessment through the school. Its small child-study team thought a reading disability highly unlikely in Luke's case, since he had made it to seventh grade without being tagged by a teacher for testing. The specialist's body language clearly reflected her opinion that we were behaving like helicopter parents overly engaged in our son's life. She reluctantly agreed to test Luke, however, and she made an appointment for us to return in a few days. When we arrived, she reported that, by her observations, Luke could read very well, and that he was "lazy and manipulative." She strongly suggested that we go home and "kick him in the behind" to curb those undesirable traits, because he would otherwise "try to get away with whatever he could."

Was she kidding? How could she not have seen what was clearly evident to us? Was I crazy? Mark witnessed the same problem—was he crazy also? Her description of Luke as "lazy" and "manipulative" did not fit the child living in our home who so clearly wanted to succeed, but who seemed to be falling deeper into a withdrawn melancholy.

We had once again sought professional help, and once again the report didn't support the notion of a larger problem. Mark and I were confused and at odds about what Luke needed, and all three members of our little family felt tension building, with nothing definitive to explain why.

Unsupported by professional opinions, I remained unable to convince anyone else that something was wrong with Luke. The pediatrician had dismissed my concerns, as had the nursery school teacher, the school psychologist, the pediatric neurologist, the independent child psychologist, and now the school's reading specialist. Mark and I had tried the "tough love" approach, allowing Luke to suffer the consequences of his actions, so long as it didn't threaten his safety, and except when it was clear that he was simply lost. The tactic of letting him flounder had failed miserably so far, and I couldn't understand why the universal principle that actions have consequences didn't seem to register in Luke's mind. That disconnect was likely the single most confusing element of raising him.

Now, confused by the contradiction between our own observations of Luke's slow reading and the specialist's assessment that his reading abilities were normal, we were left to try to improve his skills and instill an enjoyment of reading at home. Yet the deeper into adolescence Luke grew, the more he refused our involvement. That was understandable, and perhaps a good sign of maturity, but it didn't solve his reading difficulties.

Contemplating how trying and failing time and again must feel for Luke, it became clear to me that if I were in his shoes and facing mounting failures despite trying hard, I would likely also be manipulating the world around me to hide my feelings of worthlessness. And I could only imagine how weighed-down Luke must feel at being so misunderstood.

Stones Across the Water

During the summer between seventh and eighth grade, Luke agreed to attend a sleep-away tennis camp. We found a nationally organized option within our state, and it seemed ideal for him. Housed on the campus of a private boarding high school, it was only about an hour from home, and as we dropped him off, we were hopeful he would make some friendships with kids who shared his interests. When I returned five days later to pick him up, it seemed at first glance that he was right in the mix with the other kids. But as I watched them pack and interact, it quickly became obvious that Luke was, at best, only on the periphery of that fun.

During the ride home, I tried my usual line of questioning: genuine interest in Luke's enjoyment, coupled with a poorly masked hope that he might begin to come out of his shell and form some lasting friendships. He soon dashed those hopes, however, making it clear he had been by himself for most of the week's after-tennis activities. When he described the evening at a local water park, his words pointed to only one possible conclusion: that he had spent the time there alone. My heart ached, sensing his loneliness. I tried to focus on the positive: Luke had navigated the water park on his own without getting lost and had successfully regrouped with his campmates for the trip back to the school. Granted, this park was only about a tenth the size of the amusement park from his fourth-grade missed opportunity, but still, Luke had displayed a level of maturity that should be celebrated. *The social connections will follow. Of course they will.*

At the end of Luke's annual physical later that summer, the pediatrician called me into his office and surprised me with some news: Luke wanted to attend high school at the boarding school where he had stayed during tennis camp. Luke had never mentioned it to Mark or me, but he had apparently shared his wishes with the doctor. The pediatrician encouraged the interest, and said that if we were concerned about Luke not finding success in a public school with larger class sizes, a boarding school might prove the ideal solution. He had attended one himself, and said it was the best decision he and his family could have made.

Over the next few weeks and months, the three of us held a few family discussions about the possibility of Luke attending boarding school. Knowing that admission to his particular school of interest was exceptionally selective, we also toured one that was known to be a little more relaxed. It too was only about an hour from home and, much to our delight, Luke felt even more comfortable there. We made appointments for interviews at both schools.

Wishing to keep Luke at home longer, yet wanting to honor what seemed to be his desire for more independence, we also suggested another possible option of a non-boarding boys' school about forty minutes from home. Several boys from our area applied to this school each year, and because our K-8 system had a reputation for high academic standards, many were accepted. A bus picked them up early in a neighboring town and dropped them off there in late afternoon, so despite a long day for the students, the logistics could work.

Luke prepared all three applications, but only with our help and encouragement. Despite his obvious enthusiasm when he spoke about the schools, he lacked the initiative and mental energy to accomplish his own goal by completing the paperwork, which we found both confusing and frustrating. We kept thinking he might be better served if we didn't help with the process, yet Luke's middle school social studies teacher, who had taken an interest in him, encouraged us otherwise. She thought any of these three schools would be exactly what Luke needed, and asked Mark and me to not derail the endeavor just because he had not yet matured sufficiently to take charge of the application process. She believed that once maturity caught up with Luke, it would be smooth sailing from then on. Her words were reassuring, so we did as she suggested. Like her, we instinctively knew that public high school, with its large class sizes, would not be the best fit for Luke, and that his classmates were unlikely to make high school any less painful for him than they had made middle school. He clearly needed a fresh start.

At this point, I still believed Luke's measured and recognizably high IQ would sustain him academically, so we set up Luke's first interview with the school that had housed the tennis camp. Well-known for its academic prowess, even its campus reflected an aura of excellence. The interviewer was astute, and she ascertained in Luke a dissimilitude that would preclude a good match for them. Nothing was said that day; the thin-enveloped rejection letter arrived in the mail several weeks later.

Chillingly, I still recall the interview Mark and I shared with her following her conversation with Luke. She made an effort to catch my eye, and I sensed she wanted to ask, "Why are you here? Your son needs help; this is not the environment for him!" She never did, of course, and I rationalized away the unease I felt in her presence. Yet her powerful glances stayed with me for a long time. In her I saw confirmation of my own concerns, but I shook off that discomfort and focused on the interviews yet to come.

The second school, which was also a boarding school, but slightly less academically rigorous, had a more welcoming feel. Luke's interview went well, as did Mark's and mine. There was a sense of comfort here that hadn't been present at the first school.

Neither Mark nor I could imagine our child heading off to a boarding school at age fifteen, but both the pediatrician and Luke's social studies teacher strongly encouraged us to let Luke follow this path if his interest remained high. A few weeks later, a large packet from this school arrived in the mail for Luke, and I knew without opening it that he had been accepted.

I took the packet with me when I picked him up from school that afternoon, wanting to see his reaction and share a celebratory moment. He did seem happy, with his small, shy smile, but only in a muted way. His reaction to the news lacked ebullience and, knowing how he had insisted he wanted to attend boarding school, I found that disconnect perplexing.

The next interview was with the parochial boys' high school (which was not a boarding school) located several towns and one diocese away from our home. Its crisp attention to detail indicated standards of academic rigor that we were advised could spell long-term success for our son. The interviewer happened to be a physics teacher, which fit nicely with Luke's long-professed desire to become a physicist. To my relief, Luke emerged from his relatively lengthy meeting standing tall and with his sweet face reflecting an expression of pride. The teacher directed Luke to a waiting area while he escorted Mark and me into his office. There he referred to Luke's academic capabilities in glowing terms, and indicated that they might even need to create some specially devised academic challenges to match his intelligence level. Luke's admittance was all but stated on the spot.

Mark and I exited our interview hugely relieved, and I realized I had just put all my hope into this one little basket. Walking down the hallway toward the school's lobby, we found Luke staring up at the ceiling, from which hung a two-story clock pendulum. In typical form, Luke didn't acknowledge our return; instead, he turned to the physics teacher and asked if the friction of the some-part-or-other of the pendulum had been considered when it had been installed into the ceiling, and if so, how? At that, the interviewer turned to Mark and me, shrugged his shoulders, raised his eyebrows and gave us a smile that clearly said, "See what I mean?"

We envisioned success there for Luke from every angle and were relieved that he seemed comfortable at that school, despite its strict dress code and sense of formality, which Luke disliked. In truth, we weren't ready for Luke to live away from home, so when this viable and commutable option had come along, offering him the chance to not only succeed but also thrive, we were ready to jump on it if Luke's interest remained high. After that successful interview, we were unprepared for another missed opportunity, so I found myself breathless with disappointment when it presented itself in the form of a very thin envelope.

One of Luke's classmates had also applied to that school. He had no struggles academically or socially and was a wonderful all-around athlete, in addition to being a great kid. This child also received the thin envelope, startling not only his parents but us as well. We all soon learned that the school had unexpectedly limited entrance for that year to boys who lived within their own diocese. We were devastated, and it took a few days of feeling sorry for myself and for my son before I could regain my determination to find a workable and suitable path for him.

Luke had expressed a desire to attend high school anywhere but at the local public school where most of his classmates would be continuing on, so we made peace with this defeat, refocused, and looked toward the three remaining local options. Two were boys' parochial schools, and the third was a private co-ed high school promising academic rigor, but lacking organized social activities. Luke went through the interview process at the co-ed school, but since it lacked any social or extracurricular activities, I was relieved when he crossed it off the list.

That left only the two local boys' parochial schools as alternatives to the boarding school. Interviews were not required, but we did attend their open houses. In each case, there was a disproportionate emphasis on sports over academics. My heart sank deeper, but I consciously glued on a smile through the process while Luke tried to find his niche. My outward mien was entirely at odds with my inner turmoil, and I thought Luke must surely have detected my false enthusiasm. He remained silent after touring both schools, and Mark and I were left to guess which way he was leaning.

Luke's eighth-grade spring break arrived soon after, and we planned a vacation near a large saltwater sound. Luke was drawn to natural beauty, and we often traveled to spend time along the water's edge.

On one trip when Luke was younger, we had found a beautiful little lake. Mark picked up a stone and skipped it across the top of the water. The ripples that resulted delighted Luke. Mark, taking advantage of an opening to connect with his young son, showed him how to find the flattest stones and then how to hold and sidearm them so they would skim across the water's surface. Luke learned that skill fairly easily, and we had many contests over the years to see which of us could skip a stone the most times and whose stone could create the best ripples.

Now, though, adolescent Luke was especially withdrawn and visibly sad. School was not going well for him, and he had begun to realize he bore the brunt of schoolyard jokes. We walked to the water's edge and began our familiar family game. Luke didn't have his heart in it, and although he gave a semblance of trying, his stones immediately sank.

The three of us sat quietly, watching the ripples flow out and away from the sinking stones. A thought suddenly came to mind, and I looked over at Luke. I mentioned that those ripples reminded me of how quickly and how far words and actions, both good and bad, reach. It began a conversation that I hope to always remember.

Luke listened as Mark and I shared with him some examples of those far-reaching effects: how an unexpected smile from a stranger might bring a smile to our own faces; how someone could tell a lie and, in so doing, damage another's reputation—and how one person's judgment of another can have expansive and devastating repercussions. We talked about how Luke's grandma had warned me strongly against the perils of judging people, which she would say was impossible unless we "walked in the other's shoes." Luke seemed to relax a bit, and over the next few years, when he would seem especially down, I would look over at him and say, "Just some stones across the water, dear."

Years later, that phrase would take on an additional meaning. Medical, psychological, and educational professionals' failure to identify and treat what would soon be diagnosed as Luke's brain injury, combined with the judgment of family and friends that his problems seemed to be the result of bad parenting or Luke's own innate flaws, created a ripple effect so widespread and encompassing that it eventually consumed him. Stones across the water that would cost our beloved son his life.

All But Two

On the flight home from that trip, Mark asked Luke if he'd decided where he wanted to attend high school. Luke had obviously given this some thought, because his answer came quickly, with just a hint of self-doubt and hesitation: "I'm not quite ready to sleep away from home." He went on to say he'd like to attend one of the local parochial boys' schools, adding that he hoped to switch to the boarding school for sophomore year. The local option was not a great fit for Luke, and Mark and I both knew it, but we celebrated the relief that he would remain home with us for a while longer.

A few weeks later, I invited a friend to join me for an all-day outing beginning at eight o'clock in the morning. After getting permission from the school to drop her two children and Luke at the school fifteen minutes earlier than normally allowed, I made arrangements to pick up the other family at 7:40 and threw a basketball in the trunk so our kids would have something to do while they waited for the others to arrive.

My friend emerged from her house that morning with only one of her children in tow, a daughter three or four years younger than Luke. She told me that her son—a popular football player—didn't want to go with us that morning because he would have had nothing to do while he waited for his friends to arrive. I mentioned the basketball that was in the car, but she repeated that her son had said he would have no one to hang out with until his friends showed up.

A few sentences into her explanation, I tapped her on the knee and indicated Luke was sitting in the back seat, presumably listening.

Although unhappy about the early departure, Luke had been looking forward to playing basketball with her son. She turned and said hello to Luke, then continued her saga about why her son had decided not to come with us since he felt there would have been "nothing for him to do," and so she had arranged a ride to school with one of his buddies. Her voice was higher-pitched than usual, and she appeared embarrassed and uneasy. Luke's face in the rearview mirror looked pale. Had he fully realized it sounded as though her son (and she by compliance) considered him invisible—or was he simply tired?

When we arrived at the school, my friend whisked her daughter into the building, saying the girl had a meeting with a teacher. It wasn't until later that I suspected she hadn't wanted to leave her daughter with Luke. *Why?* Even with Luke's prickly behavior as of late, there was never a question of him being a danger in any way.

I was crushed for Luke. As I waited for my friend to emerge from the school, thoughts rattled in my brain. I had two choices. If I canceled the plans for the day and "rescued" Luke, he would realize that the conversation in the car had been about him, and he would be faced with the knowledge that it seemed this woman and her children had deliberately shunned him. The other option was to leave him on his own to wait for other kids to arrive at the school as if nothing was wrong. With that choice, at least there was a slim hope that Luke hadn't processed her words in the way she had by all outward appearances intended.

I made the choice to leave him standing there alone, hoping that he had escaped the full impact of her words and of her son's absence, but I never knew for sure.

Eighth-grade graduation was a reprieve for Luke; he had experienced more than his share of ego bruising from classmates, parents, teachers, and parent coaches during his nine years at this school. Graduation meant graduation parties, and the school had a policy that invitations could only be distributed on school grounds if every classmate was included. Two families chose to ignore that policy, and each excluded the same two children: Luke, and another child who had received remedial help throughout his years at this school.

One of Luke's friends told him everyone was invited, and Luke asked us what he should do since he didn't have an invitation. We knew he had only a few friends at this school, but nothing about his immaturity and lagging social skills seemed cause for shunning; certainly his teachers and school administrators had brought nothing serious to our attention. Almost every other child in his class had found a niche over the years and had come to fit in with a social group, if only on the periphery; but Luke had only one or two classmates he could remotely call his friends. Being shunned from two mostly inclusive parties would certainly add damage to his already challenged psyche. Mark knew one of the party-hosting families well enough to call and directly address the issue. He spoke with the mother, who simply retorted that her daughter could invite anyone she wished, and she had chosen to not invite Luke. I can still recall the look on Luke's face when he realized he had been deliberately excluded.

This shunning shook Mark and me along with Luke. Had there been any doubt before, Mark and I now fully understood why our son had decided to attend high school anywhere but with these classmates. A wise decision indeed.

High School, One Two Three

The local parochial high school required the boys to wear button-down shirts and ties to class, and Luke, although happier in jeans and tee shirts, accepted those terms begrudgingly. At first, he took the bus to school, and many times I would find myself out walking the dog in the afternoons when he was due home. It provided an opportunity to gauge by Luke's stride as he walked the two blocks home from the bus stop how well the day had gone. In elementary school, Luke, socially clueless in so many ways, had nonetheless maintained an exuberant and enthusiastic spirit. Those bursts of glee had leveled off in middle school, and I was hoping high school would provide a chance for him to make new friends and to feel a sense of belonging. I looked for encouraging signs in his body language, but watching him walk toward me after school brought only one word to mind: fatigue. *Why would school so visibly exhaust a fifteen-year-old boy?*

After a few months, recognizing that the school bus took a circuitous route that doubled travel time to an hour, I asked Luke if he would like me to drive him. He said yes, but unfortunately, as weeks turned into months, these rides turned into mostly unpleasant experiences. Luke became more defiant and rude as his fatigue and failures escalated. Often, wanting him to get to school on time and with a low level of stress, I chose to ignore his rants, since it seemed to me that he was angry at the world in general and that letting off steam might be therapeutic somehow.

One morning, Luke crossed a behavioral line that I couldn't tolerate and I pulled the car into a side street and stopped. He looked stunned and then resumed hollering, despite my terse explanation as to why the car wasn't moving. Five minutes passed. Finally he wore himself out long enough to take a good breath, at which point I jumped in to tell him he had a choice: he could apologize and we could continue these trips to school for as long as he maintained respect, or else this would be his last ride to school, and he would go back to taking the bus. He looked at me with an expression of confusion, managed an apology, and impulsively started to yell again. By then, the car was already back on the road and heading toward the school, and all I wanted to do was get Luke to school and use the quiet of the drive home to de-stress. At my wit's end, I dropped him at school ten minutes late, and called after him to make sure his enrollment in the bus program was still in effect.

After a month-long hiatus, I began driving Luke again periodically, hoping once again for opportunities to talk and deepen our bond. We did have some good conversations—not always pleasant, but often eye-opening, and whenever he grew sullen and yelled at me, I turned the anger inward for initiating the rides to school in the first place. At the same time, I was desperate to get at the root of his frustration, and I hoped to learn through our conversations at least some of what Luke might need. The one thing I took away from our talks was the depth of his unhappiness, but unfortunately its source remained a mystery. He had by then become a master of deflection and deception.

That Luke carried a burden was obvious; how to pull it to the surface to deal with it was not. One day it dawned on me that, because Luke had basically given up reading, he had missed the entertainment of the popular wizard Harry Potter. The audio version of the first book had just been published, and an idea hatched. It was late fall, so darkness set in early. What little homework Luke had was done, so right after dinner, with Mark out of town, I led Luke into our darkened family room with the promise of a surprise. Earlier that day I had set out a tray of candles and had inserted the first CD into the player, so it didn't take long to set the stage, bringing a much-needed smile to Luke's face. From the first introductory words to the final, dramatic sentence, the magic of the story unfolded in our ears, one or two CDs each night.

Luke never missed a beat, never lost focus, and seemed to take in even minor details from the versatile action in the narrator's voice. Not only was it a week of sweet memories for me, it was also an epiphany. Luke appeared to learn very well through audible input, much better than if he had tried to read the book himself. The two of us talked about the story after each CD ended, and Luke's precise and enthusiastic recollections surprised and encouraged me. I hadn't planned it this way, but the only sound in the room was the narrator's voice, and with the lights turned off, there were no other distractions to interfere with his auditory intake. The obvious takeaway from the experiment was that listening to a book seemed a good way for Luke to learn. From that point on, I tried to advocate for Luke to sit in the front of the classroom, or to receive assignments using audible learning materials. But without a real diagnosis of any kind, those requests to Luke's teachers were almost completely ignored.

Luke came home every day that school year more and more dejected, and by early spring he revisited the topic of the boarding school. This time the tone of his voice held an intensity that had been lacking the previous year. He clearly was unhappy with the thought of staying at his current high school and seemed desperate to make a change. Combative words weren't uncommon for Luke post-puberty, but since he normally didn't seem angry in a focused way, I had learned to look the other way, realizing he sounded more chafed than he really was. This time his words matched his demeanor, and he was visibly upset. We agreed to help him, and were thankful that the reapplication process was considerably more streamlined than the initial packet had been. Mark sat next to Luke to prompt him in making the phone call to the school to request the paperwork. And then, when the forms arrived, he sat nearby as Luke laboriously filled in the blanks. Despite Luke's ardent claim that he did want to transfer schools that fall, he continued to need reminders and encouragement to focus his efforts, and to prepare and mail the forms by the deadline. It fell on us to decide if we should enable him or let him fail.

This "should we or shouldn't we" dilemma relative to Luke's schooling highlights the confusion Mark and I faced at almost every turn. Under more normal circumstances, with a different child, we would have allowed that deadline to pass, assuming if our teenager truly wanted this as badly as he claimed, he would follow through to make it happen. We would have provided a few reminders, but we wouldn't have been on top of the process, helping him through it every step of the way. If the deadline passed and the forms weren't submitted in time, oh, well. Life lesson learned the hard way.

We weren't quite one year beyond Luke's social studies teacher's latest recommendation to not let Luke fall through the cracks by allowing the application deadline to pass. If Luke did attend the boarding school, neither Mark nor I would be there to help him. That might provide opportunity enough for connecting those actions-to-consequences dots, especially since he would be a little older and hopefully more mature. So intuition told us it was okay to keep helping Luke until he "got it." Continuing to attend a school that caused him such distress, or transferring to the public school and facing the same difficulties he had endured in elementary and middle school, could spell disaster for him.

Once the reapplication forms were in the mail, I put our fears of boarding school aside, but still hoped against hope that Luke would somehow settle in and find a sense of belonging and emotional safety in his current high school. His grades, though not great, were decent, and he had almost made it through one school year without any major flags being raised by his teachers. He was also forging some friendships, albeit tentative ones, and had seemed to enjoy his participation on the school's golf team.

On the last day of freshman year, however, Luke stormed into the house after school and, standing straight and tall with his jaw clenched and his brows furrowed, he announced to me, "Well, I made it through. My motto was 'Get Tough or Die.'"

Although I had known Luke was unhappy, his words deeply unnerved me. I later overheard one of his new school friends talking with him about the humiliation Luke had endured from some of the teachers throughout that year. Apparently, his French teacher went as far as to call him an idiot on an almost daily basis. We had had little interaction with the school; with Luke's grades hovering at adequate, Mark and I had decided to leave well enough alone. That was a mistake, as it turned out. Luke's statement on the last day of school thrust a change of schools into the mandatory category, and we realized that the boarding school had now become the best, and only, option for Luke.

Early that summer, I encountered a young college student working in a store. I casually initiated a conversation with him that turned into a major revelation. "I flunked out of college when I was a sophomore," he said, "and my parents were so angry with me they took me to a psychiatrist." With happy enthusiasm, he went on to say the psychiatrist had diagnosed him with Attention Deficit Hyperactivity Disorder (ADHD) and had prescribed focusing medication, which he felt changed his life. With the diagnosis and treatment, he had been readmitted to the college and was now doing great in school.

I questioned him further, noting that his story held many parallels to Luke's. Then I couldn't wait to get home. Within minutes of walking in the front door, I had an appointment for Luke scheduled with a second pediatric neurologist, the first since he was six years old.

This appointment thankfully yielded results. Although the neurologist denied any connection between Luke's difficulties and the playground accident years earlier, he declared that Luke demonstrated nine and a half out of ten criteria for ADHD with a significant language-processing deficit. Here was the answer, the source of all Luke's problems—finally! I was ecstatic at the prospect of a solution at last. Nagging in the back of my mind were questions about Luke's difficulties that weren't answered by this diagnosis, but I pushed them aside. For the first time in twelve years, Luke had a diagnosis beyond "highly imaginative" or "a behavioral problem." Certainly *this* would lead to the help Luke needed.

Before the appointment ended, the doctor put his arm around Luke's shoulder, looked him in the eye, and asked him to listen to himself when he spoke to me. He told Luke that he was demonstrating "oppositional/defiant" behavior that needed to stop. I wholeheartedly agreed, of course, and asked for pointers to help resolve the issue—a typical one, he said, for kids struggling to succeed. Luke and I left the office with an enormous weight lifted from Luke's shoulders and from my own, sure that the cause of most of Luke's difficulties had finally been uncovered, and that solutions to years of hardship and disappointment were at hand.

Now came the task of researching what all this would mean for my son. I had a basic understanding of ADHD, but wanted to learn more. "Language processing deficit" was a new term for me, and I couldn't wait to find out if Luke's aversion to strong foreign language accents as a young child was somehow related to this condition. The "oppositional/defiant" label certainly fit, and I had to admit it felt good to hear this doctor recognize it in Luke, name it, and bring it to his attention. At the time, I naively presumed that this behavioral pattern would suddenly stop simply because Luke was now aware of it, as if it could be remedied simply by choice. How wrong I was!

Startled by such a definitive diagnosis after so many years, I hadn't thought of questions to ask until after we had left the doctor's office. We had been sent home with a new diagnosis and a prescription for focusing medication (to be used only during the school year), but with no clear treatment plan. Once I began to do a little research, it became clear that ADHD is not a one-size-fits-all diagnosis, and treatment varies. Each case presents a little differently, and determining whether to medicate, and if so, the type and dosage of medication, is done on a case-by-case basis. The same holds true for classroom accommodations. I came away from my research realizing that treatment for this condition is not always effective. Not all children respond well to the medications; impulsivity is not necessarily curbed; educational improvements are not always realized.

And then there was the issue of Luke's behavioral manifestations. My initial hope that he would automatically make a U-turn away from impulsive actions and outbursts and revert back to what had been his natural sweet self, simply because it was brought to his attention, was quickly dashed. Maybe there was a local, specialized behavioral counselor with a treatment plan for ADHD-related oppositional/defiant behavior. I phoned the diagnosing neurologist in search of one, but he had no leads. I asked if he could help Luke further, but was told that he was a diagnostic specialist only. So I set aside that concern for the time being and hoped Luke's conduct would automatically improve once he found success in the classroom. He was teetering on the brink of a very slippery slope of failure across the board, and this diagnosis had come just in time. *He had to turn toward safer ground. He must.*

Luke received his second acceptance to the boarding school as he had hoped, and we made plans for that fall, including taking the school's suggested materials list to the shopping mall. Luke overrode his dislike of shopping and managed to help me without much opposition. We completed the errand quickly and ended our outing with his choice of a fast-food lunch stop. Fast food had become a common compromise for us. Sharing a meal with Luke at this point was a challenge. I longed for open, honest communication with him, but I had no idea how to break down the emotional barriers that seemed to separate us. Trying too hard generally ended badly, but I was uncomfortable remaining totally silent. Fast-food stops made the awkwardness briefer and easier for both of us and allowed me to defer worry to another time.

During the ride home from dropping Luke at the boarding school to begin his sophomore year, I was overwhelmed by an unexpected sadness. The tears flowed so freely that I kept my face turned toward the window so Mark wouldn't see them. I had thought this would be a happy day filled with hope and promise for our son. But reality is reality, and my heart knew we had just witnessed a boy very much out of his element.

The school had planned an entire day of fun for the new students, which included water-balloon fights, tugs-of-war, and three-legged races. Wearing his yellow school tee shirt, Luke blended in well with all the other new kids, yet he lagged a few steps behind in each activity. His advisor, a young family man with a couple of toddlers and a great sense of humor, kept everyone in the mix by playing along. He seemed an ideal role model, and it was reassuring to know that Luke had taken to him through the previous interview sessions.

As I watched Luke with the other students that day, it became obvious that "disconnected" remained my son's defining characteristic. Luke participated with the others, but on the edges. *Was he simply shy?* No, it was more than that. *Was it his growing lack of confidence, an unease that had taken on a life of its own in elementary school and freshman year, that now seemed entrenched?* I wasn't sure. I knew he remained uncomfortable in my company, but I had assumed socializing with peers would be fun for him. Nothing I witnessed that day indicated comfort for Luke at any level.

Once home, I retreated to our bedroom, curled up, and sobbed. It was not that we were facing an empty nest; I never had designs on holding Luke back. Healthy independence is, after all, the endgame of raising children. I had been physically delayed in my own path to autonomy because of enduring side effects from my serious childhood illness, so I appreciated its importance. No, I wasn't sad because Luke had moved out of our home to attend school; I was sad because I had just witnessed the other new students laughing and interacting together so easily, while

Luke remained on the periphery of that fun and social connection. My heart ached for him.

I made an appointment to see the student services director regarding Luke's recent diagnosis of ADHD. Armed with the prescribed focusing medication and written instructions from the neurologist that Luke be exempt from a foreign language requirement, I had assumed this would be a simple and straightforward accommodations request. The neurologist had assured me that an ADHD diagnosis was fairly well accepted and understood by educators by this time, and that the language processing component that made learning a foreign language difficult was a fairly common partner to the diagnosis. According to him, we should have no problem getting the school to waive this requirement for Luke, so I was not prepared for what I encountered.

Because this was a private school, it was able to operate under a different set of standards than those set by the state for public education. It maintained strong academic rigor and was designed for students preparing to attend college. Class sizes were small, and class offerings were varied and challenging. But because Luke did not yet have a diagnosis when we were assessing the strengths and weaknesses of the school, we never thought to research its philosophy on accommodations for special needs.

The student services director apparently found my request to waive Luke's foreign language requirement ludicrous; he shut down the idea and told me his decision was nonnegotiable. To complicate matters further, Luke's medication would need to be held at the office of the school nurse, a ten-minute walk across campus from the dorms and classrooms. With the medication out of sight, he would have to remind himself not only to take the medicine but also to factor in extra time each morning to walk to the medical center to retrieve it. Although the medication policy made sense as a safety issue, it would present a challenge for Luke.

As Luke had grown older, he had become aware of his "differences," and he hated them. I knew he would want to keep his diagnosis a secret from this new set of peers. What's more, he struggled to wake up in the mornings under the best of circumstances, and just getting to classes on time was difficult for him. It was hard to imagine him allotting extra time to go to the nurse's office before class every day, but I rationalized that maybe his motivation to succeed would outweigh his ever-present fatigue, his lack of focus, and his need to be like the other kids. Or maybe not—because as it turned out, Luke mostly left the medication sitting alone and untouched on the nurse's shelf for the entire school year.

In spite of these setbacks, he managed to stay afloat academically that year. We did receive phone reports, mostly during the spring semester, that he was not participating in group projects, often failed to turn in homework, and did not come to class prepared with a notebook, textbook, or pen. Because there was a small student-to-teacher ratio, the teachers also noticed fairly quickly that Luke took no notes in class. None. Handwriting had always been difficult for him, but I had naively hoped that the process of note-taking would exercise the skill and provide the remedy. Instead, he almost never set pen to paper. With only ten or so students in a class, however, distractions were minimal and Luke was able to retain the information being taught just by listening. So he got by, and our blind optimism for his future somehow managed to endure.

Dorm life presented issues for Luke as well. Like the academic advisor, the dorm supervisor was also a great role model. Fun and easy-going, he demanded only some degree of organization and cleanliness from each student. Luke's dorm room was often deemed "unsatisfactory," but in spite of losing privileges as a result, he didn't correct his mistakes. The advisor was as confused as we were about why Luke didn't seem to make the connection that by not following the lenient "cleanliness" rules, he was hurting his opportunities for fun with friends. The chores were simple and quick, and the rewards for doing them were well worth the effort. Technically Luke could handle the work, but when would he begin to initiate efforts to choose fun over penalty?

Luke was accepted onto the school's golf team that fall, providing an opportunity to develop his confidence and self-assurance. Mark and I often traveled to watch him play, and we were delighted to witness his demeanor on the course. If Luke could take charge of focusing and doing well on the golf course, didn't it follow that he would also begin to focus better academically?

And then in midwinter, we learned that he had taken an interest in a new sport: shot put. He took to it so well that he became a lead thrower on the JV team. Success with shot put provided another boost of confidence for Luke, and I can easily recall the growing sense of calm and hope I felt for my son. I wanted so badly for him to find paths that would lead him to a successful, happy life.

Yet even as he flourished in this new sport, Luke's behavioral and social development retained glaring gaps. Whenever we arrived for the track-and-field events, he completely ignored us. This leap from silence and contrariness to snubbing us altogether was both unexpected and, by any measure, rude. I might have expected such behavior during his middle school years, but not at this age. If this was maturity finally settling in, its evolutionary process seemed far from ideal.

Early the following spring, Mark was outside doing yard work when a couple drove by looking to buy a home in our cul-de-sac. Although our house wasn't on the market, they presented a more than fair cash offer, prompting us to consider if a change of venue might be just what we needed. Living in that community and witnessing difficulties and hurt for our son at every turn had taken its toll. Recognizing the gift we had just been handed, we welcomed this unexpected opportunity.

In short order, we found a lovely college town with good commuter options for Mark and a home we were both drawn to immediately. By early July, we were settled in. Mark's commute by train, although slightly longer than the bus ride had been, was more amenable to reading, a plus for him. Luke's school was now only thirty minutes away by back roads instead of an hour on highways—another plus. Even Luke, resistant to change of any kind, seemed to adapt easily enough to our new home and new town.

Within several days of our midsummer move, a radio advertisement by a national company claiming to remediate reading disabilities through innovative testing and treatment caught my attention. Intrigued, I found that it was a highly rated and successful program. The closest office was over an hour away, but after calling and asking abundant questions, I found both their tactics and their answers sufficiently encouraging to make the effort. At the very least, I reasoned, they could do no harm, and I made an appointment for Luke to undergo a full morning of evaluative testing. Although it was a hot summer day and Luke would have preferred to sleep in, he offered little resistance once I mentioned this was an opportunity to improve his reading skills.

After Luke completed the tests, the clinician called me into her office to review his results. She indicated points of success and of generalized weakness, then looked up from the paperwork and hesitated for a moment or two. Her face took on a concerned expression as she began to explain the significance of one test in which Luke's scores were startlingly low. The test measured "concept imagery," and because Luke scored only in the second percentile, she and her colleagues felt this highlighted a weakness that had an all-encompassing effect on his ability to read.

I didn't immediately grasp the meaning or significance of this area of deficit. The reading assessor explained with an example: "A black cat ran down a crooked road lined with green and yellow trees, and he passed a woman in a red dress." She then asked me what I "saw" when I heard that sentence. That was easy. "A black cat, a crooked road, green and yellow trees, and a woman in a red dress."

"Do you see them clearly in your mind?" she asked.

"Yes, of course."

"Well, Luke doesn't, and that's the problem." She went on to tell me that he appeared to have very little ability to visualize in his brain what he read, and as a result, he needed to evaluate the meaning of sentences and paragraphs from the words themselves, rather than from their combinations as most successful readers do. She told me that this deficit would have a profound effect on Luke's ability to comprehend what he read, to receive and interpret written and oral information correctly, and to express his thoughts both orally and in written form. It would also affect his ability to follow multistep directions. Remediation was available through this company, but the cost was exorbitant, both in financial outlay and in time, since treatment would involve two to three sessions per week, an hour from home. Duration of treatment was described as "open-ended."

Mark and I discussed this as an option for Luke, but decided it made more sense to take these findings to Luke's school for them to devise a plan of remediation. Exhilarated with what I presumed was the finally uncovered true source of Luke's reading challenges, I set up an appointment with the student services director. The test results explained clearly why Luke, despite having a large vocabulary and the ability to read individual words easily, struggled with reading comprehension and therefore reading speed. He had to expend an inordinate effort trying to tie all the words together to provide meaning, when that process for most people is simplified by mental visualization. Surely, this request would be openly received and an appropriate plan of remediation immediately instituted for Luke by the start of junior year.

Instead, the director of student services downplayed the findings. He explained that any serious reading weakness would have been discovered in elementary or middle school, and suggested the company that had performed the test was perhaps manipulating results to gain students and thereby income. As a parent wanting the best for my child, I recognized I could be easy prey for such a ploy, and didn't actually know how to categorize the information I had been given from either source. Luke was doing okay at this school so far. With that bird in hand, I chose to believe the student services coordinator and to let go of the reading test outcome, accepting that my desperation made me ripe for financial manipulation.

This is another point at which I wish I had taken a stronger, more confident stand. Those findings on the reading evaluation described Luke's difficulties to a tee, and the problems the assessor described as likely results of his deficit were actually happening to Luke on a daily basis. Concept imagery weakness would logically affect all areas of language processing and communication, including, or maybe especially, reading. How I wish I had not dropped that ball and had found some kind of remediation for that weakness.

Instead, I rationalized that a good education was the bottom line. I was hopeful that Luke's teachers would provide remediation for him as soon as that need became more apparent to them. Luke had been able to hide his reading problems in the past, but with so few students in the classroom and a heads-up from the services director, they would, I believed, become obvious. I looked the student services coordinator directly in the eyes and asked him to provide a copy of this latest test to all of Luke's teachers. He agreed, and I believed him. Once the teachers saw this report, they would naturally devise a plan to help Luke. It never dawned on me that a school with an excellent reputation for high standards would ignore a student's learning disability. It simply never dawned on me.

Junior year began on September 10, 2001, and Luke seemed happy to return to the boarding school. The events of the following day raised our country's collective consciousness, and Luke was no exception. By nature sensitive and kindhearted, he was strongly affected by the attacks on our country that resulted in the deaths of so many innocent people. Mark was in New York and scheduled to be at the World Trade Center that day, for lunch as it turned out, so I got word to Luke as quickly as I could that his dad was okay.

This was also Luke's first year to study physics, and he had been anticipating that all summer. His interest in the subject had remained strong for many years, and his intention to become a physicist had never waned. Over the summer, Mark had read Stephen Hawking's *A Brief History of Time* to Luke, and the two engaged in animated conversation about its content after each chapter ended. Luke was clearly anxious to get his study of physics underway.

By the time parents' weekend arrived in mid-October, however, Luke appeared more distracted than ever, and we had already begun receiving calls from his teachers. After just a few weeks of school, Luke had apparently "quit." He spent his time tossing a Frisbee alone on the quad, and he rarely showed up for class. Luke's advisor and his teachers assumed his reaction to the 9/11 attacks had derailed him. It indeed had a strong impact, but there was also another cause for his disconnect from school.

We knew that Luke's physics teacher was a recent immigrant to the United States, and that she spoke with a strong foreign accent. I recalled how Luke as a little boy had shied away from anyone with a foreign accent, and now I understood that the "language processing" component of the ADHD diagnosis, intertwined with his newly uncovered concept imagery deficit, was the likely reason. Upon learning of the teacher's language barrier at the start of the school year, I had contacted the student services representative, but to no avail. He told me that the other children were acclimating to the strong accent and that Luke needed to learn to adjust as well. He emphasized it was Luke's responsibility to adapt to school policy, not the school's to adapt to Luke.

So when Mark and I attended parents' weekend, the first class we visited was Physics. Neither of us could decipher a word the foreign-born teacher spoke, and with heavy hearts, we understood why our son was spending his time anywhere but in the classroom. Having looked forward to studying physics for so long, Luke found his hopes shattered. Unable to understand the teacher's words, he simply gave up. To make matters worse, Luke was led to believe it was his fault, judging from the remarks by the student services representative.

Luke needed to get back in the game immediately and fully if he were to have any chance of recouping the semester. Mark and I took him to a local restaurant for dinner that evening, and the conversation proved interesting. We discussed his options, including leaving the boarding school (knowing he would be asked to leave soon unless he made a quick turnaround) and transferring to the local high school in our new town. To our surprise, Luke not only engaged in the discussion, but also made the decision to come back home and transfer to the public high school in our new district. He actually seemed relieved at the prospect.

So, on November 1 of his junior year, Luke began attending his third high school in as many years. He knew only one classmate, an outgoing kid whom he had met on the golf course during the preceding summer. This fellow went out of his way to introduce Luke to his friends and to acclimate him to the school. Unfortunately, Luke eventually indicated to us that he had little in common with this guy and his friends, despite my hope to the contrary. Luke was a confusing combination of a type B, laid-back personality and alternative-music-loving, defiant and impulsive young man. Most of the students he was introduced to were highly focused and successful, vying for admission to the best colleges and universities, and were strongly motivated, competitive kids. Luke, unable to compete in the classroom, attracted and was attracted to students who, either by nature or their life histories, shied away from competition as he did. As Luke watched the successful, competitive students glide toward their goals, he became only more defiant and withdrawn.

Lion and Lamb

The memories that follow continue to take my breath away. It felt, as they were happening, as if the safety and success we had wished for our son and had assumed were always just around the corner were suddenly tossed into the grip of a hurricane. We had no control over the direction it took or the devastation it caused. We could only look on and watch it happen.

As Luke immersed himself in this new school, he became more and more social, often inviting friends to our house. That was the good news of the transfer. Some of the kids were polite and adorable late bloomers, while others set off warning bells in my head. I tried to have conversations with Luke about making good social choices, but he just pulled further and further away from a middle ground. He began to push curfew past its limits, and he took on a level of defiance that overrode even his "Get Tough or Die" motto from several years earlier. His eyes took on a glazed appearance that even this drug-ignorant mother could not ignore. I couldn't find evidence to ground my theory, but all the signs indicated Luke was using drugs of some kind.

Now more than ever, Luke needed our help. Although we had certainly warned him over the course of years about the dangers of using illegal drugs and alcohol, he had apparently fallen prey to them. I went to work at reading everything I could get my hands on about teens and substance abuse, but application of this new knowledge failed. Luke was still a babe in the woods in so many ways, remaining disconnected to the concept that actions have consequences. To make matters worse, whatever substance was clouding his eyes was also elevating his outbursts. What had been difficult flare-ups since middle school now became unmanageable eruptions of anger and frustration.

I didn't know what to do about Luke's newly discovered and suddenly active social life, so I put my head in the sand and rationalized that most of Luke's friends seemed to be kids you would want your son to bring home. None were compulsively focused, straight-A students, but most were doing just fine. I hoped and prayed the few whose own eyes were glazed over would soon fall off Luke's radar. I became hypervigilant, but my ignorance and minimal efforts were not enough to guide Luke to a safer path. Mark seemed far less concerned, and I leaned on his calmness to help balance my fears.

When the second semester began in January, many of Luke's teachers began calling, although infrequently at first. His guidance counselor questioned on several occasions if Luke would be better off in a private school with smaller class sizes. I explained each time that we had already gone that route, and because the boarding school did not make accommodations for students with learning differences, it had not worked for him. I asked her for recommendations of other private schools that might be a better fit, but she did not know of any. She did set up a meeting with the high school's child study team, and through them a Section 504 accommodations plan was formulated for Luke, based on the ADHD diagnosis. He was less than compliant, however, and balked at sitting in the front of the classroom, or having another student take notes for him, or taking his tests separately. In a moment of willing conversation, he told me that he was finally comfortable socially in this school and wanted to be "one of the guys"; he didn't want to be "different." It was understandable from the point of view of a teenager, but at the same time, Luke's adamant refusals closed doors to opportunities for his education. Luke was aware of the ADHD diagnosis, but its significance and the importance of those classroom accommodations eluded him. We'd yet to find a replacement for the diagnosing neurologist from our old town, and because the daily dose of ADHD medication that Luke was now taking was not working, the two psychologists whom we took Luke to see would not renew the prescription, opting instead to treat him with "talk therapy."

According to the teachers' calls, Luke was quickly "lost" in the throng of thirty or more kids in a classroom, and his ability to "listen to learn" was severely compromised by the distractions and extraneous sounds of a packed room. And although by this time I had forgotten about the "noise of five TVs going at once" inside Luke's head, I later learned that the barrage had continued unabated for all those years, compromising not only his ability to absorb information in a large, noisy classroom, but also his ability to feel comfortable and calm in his own skin.

By early spring of his junior year, calls were coming in from most of Luke's teachers on an almost daily basis. I came to dread the sound of the phone ringing, but kept promising these caring professionals that we would continue to work with Luke on organizational skills (making sure his books and supplies went with him to school) and on responsibilities (completing homework assignments and studying). The messages became increasingly dire; Luke's teachers were universally concerned that Luke kept his head on his desk throughout class, appearing totally disengaged. Like me, however, they clung to hope simply because he kept showing up for class.

To make matters worse, Luke became increasingly secretive and withdrawn as the school year progressed. My own adolescence hadn't been accompanied by this level of what I assumed was teen angst, but every person is different, and I didn't want to overreact. At the same time, though, there was no way as a parent I could allow Luke to get away with not participating at school or being disrespectful at home without significant consequences, natural and otherwise.

Mark remained confused and understandably angered by our son's choices, and I floundered trying to figure out how to best handle Luke's verbal outbursts, which seemed to worsen day by day, week by week.

Despite the stack of parenting books at my fingertips, none of the advice seemed to fit. What I tried, failed. I aimed for consistency; everything I read told me that eventually the consequences would be felt, and the lesson would be learned. This still did not work for Luke, and I sank only deeper as I tried to understand why.

My goal was to stand in what I thought was Luke's corner, rife with love and encouragement, but also with plenty of consequences for undesirable choices. Luke saw me as the enemy in a way that, taken alone, I might have mistaken for normal adolescent growing pains. But Luke's attitude pushed all boundaries of acceptability. Continuing to make no connection between his actions and the consequences that followed, he only became increasingly angry with me for imposing those consequences. I disconnected his cell phone for periods of time and grounded him as immediate and relative results of specific bad choices. It wasn't unusual for our car to turn around and go back home if Luke was disrespectful while he rode with me to his tennis lessons. Despite thinking that exercise was beneficial for Luke, eventually we even canceled those lessons entirely. But at the same time, trying to catch Luke doing anything positive became a daily, if not hourly, goal. Why wasn't Luke showing some signs, any sign, to indicate he was figuring out how to make life work in his favor? I was so disheartened and frantic for his immediate and future well-being that the only relief from worry came with sleep at the end of the day.

Frustratingly, these attempts at enforcement, both negative and positive, had little impact on him. Of course, he disliked the negative and would have preferred a pat on the back, but that preference failed to inspire him to change his actions. Instead, Luke became angry simply because there were consequences. As the at-home parent, I was usually the target for his anger. Interestingly enough, moments after shouting at me, Luke would often appear perfectly calm, relaxed, and friendly again. My resentment of his disrespect kept bristling, however, and I avoided him for a period of time afterward. His ability to so quickly forget his foul behavior only added fuel to my irritation, and I was often stunned by his inability to understand why. Luke's outbursts were especially confusing as they seemed aimed into the space around me, rather than directly at me. His eyes didn't make contact with mine, and his emotional discomfort was all-encompassing, diluting his efforts to make his point. He would yell at the space above my head in rage—but he had difficulty making a clear and concise point relative to the topic.

Luke and I were making it through our days misaligned and unable to match our desires for good communication with our responses. Whenever Luke was ill or otherwise uncomfortable, though, an amazing transformation occurred. He would become childlike, welcoming my nurturing tendencies, whether they came in the form of a hot cup of tea or a kiss on his forehead. Invariably, in the sweetest reversion to the child he had been, he would bring on that little smile that so endeared him to me, and say softly, "Thanks, Mom."

I loved those moments, and knew the child in him was still very much there, inside this young adult's body. They helped me believe that his sometimes raging and seemingly irrational anger was actually the child within him reacting to fear and frustration. I just didn't know why. How I longed to see authentic snippets of maturity taking hold. As adorable as these childlike moments were, they weren't indicative of the "normal" and age-appropriate developmental track I hoped he would find.

My heart also ached for Mark as he watched his son's chances for success disintegrate before his eyes, powerless to turn him around. He had grown tired from having no road map to help lead his son off the sticky path of looming failure. We were both in way over our heads. The more Luke's failures mounted, the deeper our concern and confusion ran, and the more frustrated we became with him and with each other.

In the midst of this escalating angst within our family, Luke, who had a junior driver's license, went out one Saturday night and missed his state-imposed curfew. I was awake waiting for him to return home and trying to keep my escalating worry at bay when the phone rang. I felt immediate relief upon hearing Luke's voice, but only half believed him when he told me he had a flat tire and would be late getting home.

"Do you need any help, Luke?"

"No. I can fix it, I think."

"Well, thanks for letting us know and please call if you want Dad to meet you. It's harder to fix a tire in the dark."

"Okay, Mom. I'll be fine." And he quickly hung up before I could say another word.

I made a cup of tea and began to pace. *Was Luke telling the truth? Or was he making up a story to cover his real tracks?* I hated not trusting my own son. But Luke had learned to lie and to cover his failures with bad behavior when he was younger, and by this point he had mastered the skill. Worry morphed into fear of the unknown when an hour passed and there was still no sign of him.

The phone rang again, and I ran to pick it up. I thought it would be Luke, but when the voice on the other end was not my son's, I felt a sudden surge of panic.

The caller identified himself as a county police officer, and my heart jumped. *Where was Luke? Had he been arrested? Was he injured somewhere?* I experienced for the first time what I can only describe as an out-of-body response as the fear, heightened by years of confusion and the downward spiral surrounding Luke's emotional, social, and academic development, seemed to momentarily separate body from brain. Fortunately, this officer, sensing my anguish, quickly explained that Luke was fine, and he wanted only to let us know that our son would be late because he was changing a flat tire. To that he quickly added that Luke wasn't in any trouble for missing the curfew. Happy to know Luke was okay and that he had told us the truth, I breathed a sigh of relief as my body and brain realigned.

Luke had no problem making the golf team that spring, and his participation gave us hope that he would continue to keep his head above water socially. Respect and honesty are inherent in the sport, which offered Mark and me a welcome opportunity to have those all-important life skills reinforced.

With Luke doing well for those few weeks, I relaxed into a false sense of calm. I was certain the worst was over and that emotional and educational safety were finally within his reach. I wanted so badly to believe that. But then one day he came home from an after-school match earlier than expected, surprising me with the news that he had quit the team. He ignored my questions and disappeared into his room without explanation. But his glazed-over eyes told the tale and set me reeling once again.

Later that evening, Luke's guidance counselor called to inform us that Luke had been kicked off the team for shouting obscenities at passersby during the match. This represented a new low for Luke, and it took a few seconds for the blood to return to my head.

What neither Mark nor I realized at that moment was that this type of behavior would soon come to define our son, and that a pattern of adaptation to failure was taking hold that would spell disaster for him.

A Call for Help

One hot summer night between Luke's junior and senior year, a loud clap of thunder startled me awake. I glanced at the clock beside the bed and jumped up, realizing that Luke's curfew had long since passed. Ordinarily, on the nights when Luke was out, a good book could keep me awake until he came home, but not this time. I checked his bedroom—no one there. A quick walk through the house yielded no trace of him. Trying to stave off worry, I stood at the window and focused on the beauty of the storm, wondering what to do next. With the first light of morning approaching the horizon, there was now no escaping worry. Night had ended and Luke had not come home.

I tried calling his cell phone, but he didn't pick up. An hour later, I tried again, and then again. As the sun rose, I sent several text messages, with no reply. By midmorning, I'd called two of Luke's closest friends, but neither had seen him the evening before.

Complicating the situation was Luke's recent eighteenth birthday; he was now, for legal purposes, an adult. He was anything but an adult by measure of maturity, yet he would nonetheless need to be missing for twenty-four hours in order for us to obtain police help. For the remainder of that morning and well into the afternoon, I made calls to Luke's cell phone, but by then they went directly to voicemail. I didn't know if that meant the battery had worn down, or if Luke had turned off his phone. The latter seemed unlikely since he lived by his phone, and with that realization, my fear escalated. Four or five times that day I drove aimlessly around town, searching for Luke to no avail.

When he didn't call or return home by early evening, we finally called the police and enlisted their help. That was a terrifying moment. Officially reporting our child missing hammered home the deadly seriousness of the situation. Even with the resources of the police department, it would be another seventeen excruciating hours before we received word that Luke had been found alive in a remote corner of a parking lot in town.

A young officer escorted Luke home, sat him in a chair, and took a seat across from him. Sharply dressed in his blue uniform, he leaned toward my filthy, disheveled son, who looked as though he might fall asleep at any moment, and tried to capture his attention. In a quiet, brotherly voice, he told Luke that by choosing to stay away and not contacting us, he had placed himself in what could have been a very dangerous situation. Then he simply asked Luke why he had done it. At first Luke didn't reply, and I wondered if, bent over with his head on his folded arms, he might actually be asleep. The silence mounted for five or six seconds before Luke lifted his head and said, "Because I wanted to know what it felt like to sleep outside." And just like that, he was folded over again. As I listened to this interaction, anger welled inside me, displacing the joy I had felt with my son's safe return home. *What kind of an answer is that? At the very least, he could have called to let us know he was okay, and he could be thanking this officer for his help.* As relieved as I was to know Luke was alive and unhurt, I was also desperately frustrated with him and consumed, even more than usual, by fear and confusion.

The officer turned to me and astutely read the angst in my eyes. He then turned back to my son, who was becoming more of a stranger to me with every passing day. "Look at your mother, Luke," he said. "It will be a long time before she will fully recover from this worry." He went on to tell Luke he had a responsibility to respect his parents and himself. And then, after a long pause, he concluded in a near-whisper, "Please do not ever take that kind of risk again." If ever there was a time Luke needed to listen, it was then, and I remember digging my fingers into the arms of my chair, trying to will his brain, through any means possible, to receive that message.

But before the summer was over, Luke did take that risk again. Luckily, he was found safe for the second time. By then, I was beginning to grow emotionally numb. It seemed the only way to survive.

"Mom, I Can't Read"

In September of senior year, Luke approached me after school one day. He haltingly began a sentence, averted his eyes, and stopped talking. Rubbing his hands together self-consciously, he raised his eyes again and restarted his sentence. "Mom, I can't read."

This was a huge statement on several levels. It confirmed what Mark and I already suspected, but it also indicated that Luke's awareness of his difficulties was focusing. I tentatively prodded for more information, not wanting to upend his trust. Luckily, he continued without hesitation.

"I know all the words, but they don't fit together. I need to read paragraphs over and over again to try to make sense of them."

What he was saying didn't surprise me—though I was thrilled he had chosen to open up to me—but it did jog my memory. Until that moment, I had all but forgotten about the reading test that had seemed so important a year earlier—the one that had uncovered Luke's "concept imagery" reading deficits. The realization suddenly struck me that I had been foolish to shelve those findings despite how closely they aligned with Luke's scholastic difficulties. I had fallen prey to the suggestion that those results had been manipulated somehow as a moneymaking scheme to gain clients. None of Luke's teachers at the boarding school had mentioned reading difficulties as part of their concerns about Luke's lack of organizational skills and missing homework assignments, but surely the school's resource coordinator had shared the results of that reading test with them. Surely he had.

The messages our family received from professionals were in discord, as they had been for years, and now I had to come to terms with not only failing to address Luke's self-proclaimed academic roadblock, but also with ineffectively sorting the professional opinions along the way and knowing which to use and which to discard.

Self-loathing would have to wait. Luke needed my full attention. I asked his permission to share this news with the current school's administrators, and he reluctantly agreed. Being "different" and having problems the other kids didn't experience continued to be painful for him. Sharing his reading struggles with me suggested an awakening was finally taking place, and implied a cry for help that might override his need to be like the other kids.

I hugged him, promising to go to the school the next day, and then I watched as he walked away. His shoulders remained slumped, but I thought maybe he was standing a bit taller now that he'd been able to ask for help. It had been more than fifteen long years since the accident with the swing, and our family had been sapped of most of its recuperative resources. To say we were all floundering would be an understatement.

During those fifteen years, we had gathered piecemeal information from professionals as to the source of Luke's difficulties: the "next-Steven-Spielberg" theory, the ADHD diagnosis, and the concept imagery reading deficit. Luke had tried medication for ADHD the previous year, but the prescribed dosage hadn't seemed to help, and eventually he quit taking it. And, as difficult as it was to believe, the administrators at the boarding school had apparently discarded Luke's reading assessment. Both ADHD and the reading weakness seemed to imply a larger problem, because neither alone nor in combination did they begin to explain all of Luke's social and educational obstacles.

Lacking a diagnosis that connected all the dots, I chose unfounded optimism over rationality, clinging to the hope that Luke would eventually mature out of his failures and find success using his highly intelligent imagination. It allowed me to function. We ignored the elephant in the room that was the actual undiagnosed cause of Luke's problems. But now, suddenly, Luke had asked for help and that elephant took center stage.

The following day, I made an appointment with Luke's guidance counselor and the school's child study team. I headed into that appointment with renewed buoyancy, certain that Luke's own description of his stumbling blocks in reading comprehension would provide a path to remediation.

Appallingly, the child study team director told me the school would do nothing, despite the 504 plan already in place for him. Her response tripped off her tongue, swift and cold: "He's a senior; it's too late now." She reasoned that reading difficulties should have been uncovered and addressed in elementary school and were, therefore, not the high school's problem.

By nature I long for peace, but at that moment I wanted to pound on the woman's desk. I wanted to scream. Her refusal was unconscionable and infuriating. It was her *job* to help Luke! How could she simply pass him off as though he didn't matter? What difference did it make that this was the first time Luke could verbalize what he needed? He was saying it now, and that should matter.

I tried to remain calm. I swallowed a few times to curtail the wave of nauseating hopelessness that had begun to well up. Then, taking some preliminary deep breaths, I explained that we had tried to find help for Luke when he was in elementary school, and that I was just now realizing that they might have never tested reading comprehension, but only his ability to read aloud. The director's eyes remained hard as she repeated that there was nothing this school could or would do for Luke. With that, the meeting was over. She stood, turned, and walked into her office.

I knew this wasn't right. The school was required to assist my son; we were taxpaying residents of the district, and he was entitled to be educated there, even with special needs. The fact that an elementary school in another district hadn't detected Luke's significant reading comprehension obstacles did not let this school off the hook. He needed their help.

A few days later, Mark and I met with the school principal, but that meeting also turned out to be a waste of time. The principal barely looked up from his desk and within five minutes had ended our attempts to communicate our concerns. He had apparently predetermined the outcome of the meeting, fully supporting his team's decisions.

Mark hurried to catch a late train to work while I went home and tried to refocus my anger into energy. Opening our phone book, I found a company of reading tutors in the yellow pages and promptly set up an appointment to talk with them about Luke. If the school refused to help, we would find help somewhere else.

The tutoring company waiting room was crowded with young moms and their young children. After stepping over and around little ones to get to the reception desk, I explained Luke's needs to the receptionist and completed the required forms. That evening, the assigned tutor phoned and expressed her hesitancy to work with a student as old as Luke. "I'm used to six-year-olds," she said. "I don't think our program will work for someone as old as your son."

"Please," I begged. "Please, just allow four sessions with Luke. That's all I ask." I must have sounded pathetic. She reiterated her concerns, though in a softer tone, and then reluctantly agreed. We would have to wait a month or two before her schedule opened up, and then she would be in touch with us.

I thanked her profusely, hung up the phone, and began to cry. Tears could come easily these days whenever my thoughts landed on Luke. Tears of fear mingled with hope for his future, sadness for his past difficulties, and now frustration that even this dubious lifeline would be delayed.

While waiting for the reading tutor to call us back, I began researching other options, but could find precious few. As Luke's behavioral and academic failures compounded daily, I also turned to the specialists we had hired in the past to help: a math tutor, a literature tutor, a learning consultant, and a psychologist. One of them knew of an out-of-state residential school for at-risk boys, one with a good reputation and a history of successful outcomes. We decided we didn't have the luxury of waiting for the reading tutor to have an opening in her schedule; her help would likely not be enough to turn Luke around anyway. Mark took a vacation day, caught an early flight, and interviewed the out-of-state school, and when he returned late that evening he told me, his voice as tired as I had ever heard it, that this was at least a possibility for Luke. We were heartbroken, helpless to know what to do next for our son. It felt so much like drowning in a sea of thick air.

With disconsolate resolve, we made arrangements for Luke to transfer to the new school in January, in the hope that the professionals there could do more to help him than we had been able to do from home. But we still faced a huge hurdle: Luke would need to agree to the transfer since he was now legally an adult, and we doubted he'd cooperate. With that in mind, we kept looking for options closer to home, and every couple of weeks I checked in with the reading tutor to let her know Luke was still in need of her help.

Our search uncovered the existence of a category of professionals called educational advocates, and we bit the financial bullet and contracted with one. To anyone who has never tried, it might seem like a simple process to request educational help from a school district, but without an accurate diagnosis in hand and with the budget cuts and spending caps that school districts face, it's anything but easy. Hiring an advocate risked alienating the very people whose help we needed, but a desperate situation calls for desperate measures.

The foundation of Luke's education was, by this point, obviously cracked, its mortar missing in too many places to be sustainable. When he approached me about his reading difficulties, he, like I, anticipated that the school would swoop in to assist him. As the weeks passed with no offer of help, Luke never said anything to me about it, but his mood darkened with each empty day. He was sullen and angry over the smallest issues, which I perceived as embarrassment. I began to wonder if he also felt a degree of abandonment. Did he think I wasn't taking his request for help seriously and hadn't tried to obtain support for him? Luke's admission that he couldn't read properly, after trying to hide the problem for so long, had opened a chink in his protective armor. Now he clamped it shut again. Luke had trusted us, and in his mind, we had ignored and failed him. He wouldn't make that mistake again anytime soon.

Finally, about a month after Luke's disclosure, and armed now with the help of a paid educational advocate, we were able to arrange a second meeting with the child study team. This time, in an obvious reversal, and dancing to the tune set by our advocate, they decided more information was needed before they could determine if or how to help Luke. *More delays.* They requested a battery of educational tests and a psychiatric evaluation, which Mark and I decided to have done privately. At this point, we did not trust the school to produce unbiased results.

Meanwhile, with January fast approaching, the advocate revealed information that floored us: Luke's school already had a program in place for kids who weren't finding success in the regular classroom. I could barely contain myself. I wanted to storm into that school office and rant at anyone who would listen for needlessly putting our son, and us, through the wringer, and for delaying his chances for a viable education. Instead, I had to find the composure that was needed to fight for Luke in a workable way. Rechanneling my emotions, and with the advocate at my side, I calmly requested another appointment with the principal for the following day. Having the advocate's support made all the difference: our request was quickly granted. I decided to save mulling about the injustice of it all for another day.

We'd worked so hard for so long to secure help for Luke that at this point we would not, could not tolerate another delay. Mark took more time off from work the next morning to attend the meeting. Sitting opposite the principal, we fought back exasperation at having never been told about this program and, keeping our emotions at a simmer, asked if Luke would be a candidate for it. Aware by now that Mark and I were serious and that, given the 504 Plan already in place, maybe there really was something wrong with Luke, the principal arranged to have him transferred to those specialized classes.

We had been steeling ourselves to send Luke out of state to a new school and trust his outcome to strangers, and now, at the eleventh hour, we were able to breathe a little easier with help available practically at our doorstep. *Why had the school allowed our family's nightmare to be strung out for so long?* I couldn't take the time to think about that; there was work to be done to get Luke into a classroom setting where he just might find an opening to success.

Luke, true to form, did not fight the transfer to specialized classes. He actually seemed to look forward to them, probably because he thought they would help him learn. But within a few weeks, the glint of hope was gone from his eyes, his shy smile had all but disappeared, and his slumped body language clearly signaled that the new classes weren't working as anticipated.

As a young boy, Luke had held high hopes for his future, and his desire to do well in school had been obvious, despite his growing failures along the way. His disappointment with his introduction to physics at the boarding school had usurped much of that hope, and these alternative classes seemed to dampen what little was left. Luke told us only that the curriculum was "dumbed down," clearly frustrating his expectations.

The school gave permission for Luke to miss classes for the two days of testing they had requested at our meeting, and I couldn't help but wonder what these new tests would reveal. Standardized testing in elementary school had shown a fairly significant gap between his consistently high math scores and his inconsistent language-based scores. Luke's high IQ apparently confounded the results and made them difficult to interpret, but since his scores were high enough to pass state-mandated requirements, his teachers apparently had not addressed those discrepancies.

The outside educational examiner we hired for the school's testing requisite found similar discrepancies in Luke's scores, and, to her credit, she recognized those disparities as a learning deficit. She noted, however, that she was confused by her findings. She was trained to detect and identify classified learning disabilities, and although Luke's scores were suggestive of a problem, she could not match that problem to an already-existing classification. Still, because the testing provided indicators of difficulty, the school began to pay attention.

Next came the required psychiatric evaluation. Because Luke already had an ADHD diagnosis, I tried to locate a psychiatrist who specialized in that disorder. The learning consultant, who had been interfacing weekly with Luke's teachers on his behalf, highly recommended a physician who had written a book about children with ADHD. The book already held a prominent place on our bookshelf, so I believed an evaluation by this doctor would be fair and sound.

It was surprisingly easy to secure an appointment. The difficulty came in getting Luke there, since the doctor's office was a three-hour drive from home. My own energy was depleted, not only from accumulated worry, but also from driving Luke to so many remedial appointments each week. But Luke was willing and even a little eager to see this ADHD specialist, so we made the trip after school one evening, stayed in a motel, and spent about three hours in the doctor's office the following morning. Luke had an hour of one-on-one time with him, and then I was invited to join them to provide details and any observations that might be relevant. The physician, soft-spoken and kind, listened intently and expressed a fatherly concern toward Luke, and then personally administered several questionnaires and diagnostic tests to him. Once the testing was completed, we thanked the doctor, left his office, stopped at a nearby restaurant for a quick lunch, and headed back home. Luke fell asleep almost immediately, and didn't stir until the car turned into our driveway.

It took several weeks for the doctor to assemble the data. When we returned for the follow-up appointment, all the information had been neatly put into report format, ready to be taken to the school in compliance with their request. The psychiatrist was clear in his interpretation and support of the ADHD diagnosis, so Luke's continuation in the pullout classes seemed to make sense to everyone involved. Luke found comfort in the fact that this doctor himself had struggled with undiagnosed ADHD for many years and had been able to overcome his difficulties to become a psychiatrist and well-respected author.

"I Know What Is Wrong"

Within the next month, the private reading tutor phoned to say she had an after-school opening in her schedule for Luke. She didn't contact me after her first meeting with him, but after the second session, she phoned to tell me he needed more help than any of the six-year-olds in her care. She sounded hesitant. After several attempts to complete what was an obviously uncomfortable question, she finally blurted it out.

"Did you know Luke reads in color?"

Her question startled me to the core, not because it sounded odd, but rather because it jogged a forgotten memory: *What color are your nines, Mom?* The blood began to drain from my head. I sat down, phone in hand, and told the tutor about those colored numbers Luke had described years earlier. I could almost hear her sigh with relief as she realized her question, initially uncomfortable to say aloud, had addressed something familiar to me—and no doubt important to Luke.

Luke had explained to her that every number and letter of the alphabet had a specific and unique color overlay that was always superimposed over black lettering. The tutor wondered if perhaps Luke was fabricating, and she had tried for two weeks to trick him. She had secretly written down the colors for each letter and number he described, certain he wouldn't remember which color went with which, but Luke never missed matching the "correct" color to letter or number. "I think he's telling me the truth," she said. Sounding a bit relieved that her observations were aligned with Luke's history, she promised to look into what it all meant.

Later that week, I attended a class in watercolor painting, and mentioned this colored-letter phenomenon to one of my classmates. From across the room, another classmate who overheard the conversation exclaimed, "Oh, that's called synesthesia!"

She spelled the word for me, and as soon as I got home I looked it up and found a website that showed the color combinations exactly as Luke had described them. When Luke came home from school that afternoon I couldn't wait to show him the page I had printed out, with all the colors for each letter as he had described. He didn't seem terribly excited by it, and afterward I realized he couldn't see the page as I did, since he was unable to see it *without* the color overlays.

After the third tutoring session, the reading specialist phoned again. "I want you to take Luke to see a neurologist. I think there is something physiologically wrong with him."

I explained my hesitance, though not in detail. I had been down the physician road once too often, without benefit to Luke and with blame landing in my lap at nearly every turn. And we had the ADHD diagnosis already. What else could it be? Besides, I had described the accident with the swing to so many professionals by this point, and it hadn't seemed important to any of them. Trying with yet another would only lead to more frustration.

"Well, if you won't take him, I will," she said, and I believed she meant it.

With little hope for securing a diagnosis other than the ADHD one already in place, I located a neurologist in our new town and scheduled an appointment for Luke. Once again, I was encouraged by his eager willingness to see yet another doctor, but after dropping him at the physician's office, I mentally prepared what I might say to him when this appointment turned out to be just another exercise in futility. I returned to pick him up about half an hour later, with an undercurrent of negative thoughts rattling through my brain. Surprisingly, Luke was still in the examining room, and the physician, learning that I had arrived, came out to the waiting room to ask if I would join them.

He asked Luke's permission to speak with me. Now that Luke was over eighteen, HIPAA (Health Insurance Portability and Accountability Act) privacy laws applied, and Luke had to explicitly allow the doctor to share any of his medical information with me. Luke hesitated for a moment, then gave me one quick look as if to say "Don't mess this up" and signed the necessary paperwork.

"Please, tell me a little about Luke's history," the neurologist began.

Suddenly realizing this medical consultation had taken an interesting and hopeful turn, I tried to gather my thoughts, sifting through the years of doctor appointments, phone calls from teachers, Luke's inability to read and complete assignments, and his social difficulties. My initial impulse was to remain silent about the swing incident. In that moment I was a full-blown coward, stung too many times by physicians, educators, and family members who disregarded my concerns and told me I had overreacted to the accident by drawing a connection between it and Luke's sudden but lasting personality changes. I was exhausted by their suspicions that I was a bad mother and that Luke was a slacker. By this point, there were too many fingers pointing at both of us, and I was having trouble maintaining belief in myself—and in Luke.

Thankfully, an intuitive surge shoved those thoughts of self-pity aside. Quickly, before my mind could change, I blurted out that Luke had been struck on the side of his head prior to his third birthday and had changed dramatically from that point on.

Then, taking a deep breath, I lowered my eyes to the floor and waited for the doctor to dismiss the connection. I expected him to tell me, as all the others had, that the accident had nothing to do with Luke's difficulties. I expected that, within minutes, we would be walking out the door with only another wound to Luke's vulnerable psyche, the real cause for his escalating failures once again left undiscovered.

Instead, the doctor's words surprised and thrilled my heart:

"I know what is wrong."

Based on his examination of Luke and on the history we'd both provided, he told us he was certain Luke had sustained a closed-head traumatic brain injury when he was struck by the swing. Giving no further details, he said simply, "I'm going to send you to a cognitive neurologist, who will help you from here. Good luck with everything." He smiled and gave a nod of his head as though all would be okay, and before I knew it, Luke and I were standing together on the sidewalk outside the doctor's office.

I looked at my son, and all the years of questions and blame and frustration and failure and determination and dashed hopes and dreams crashed in on me in that one moment. Had we really just heard a physician, this neurologist, agree that the blow to Luke's head by the swing almost sixteen years earlier had caused an injury to his brain that was the source of his enduring difficulties? Was this beautiful, frustrated, depressed, persevering son of mine about to have a second chance at life? As I tried to slow my suddenly rapid breathing and to process the words we'd just heard, I reached over and grabbed Luke's arm. "Did you hear that, Luke? We've just been put on a fast track to get you all the help you need."

This doctor's short declaration was the first time anyone had connected the accident to the years of struggle that followed it. Realizing that a neurologist, trained in the workings of the human brain, had just affirmed what I had believed and feared all along, I shuddered. *What did this mean? What was a brain injury, really?* I had no idea at that moment, but I did know that somehow that strike to Luke's head had fundamentally changed my son—socially, academically, and emotionally. For the first time in sixteen years, we had a diagnosis that made sense from every angle, that connected every dot, and we had just been given a place from which to lead Luke back onto the road to a workable "normalcy." Whatever having a closed-head brain injury meant in medical terms or implied for Luke's future was unclear to me in the moment, but the diagnosis was a starting place, and the cognitive neurologist would answer all our questions and fix Luke's brain. I was certain of it.

I looked over at Luke, but his eyes were not on me. I noticed his slumped shoulders and realized that, in typical fashion, he likely had not processed the doctor's words. Luke didn't know he had just been handed the reason behind all the difficulties he had encountered up to now— the bullying and rejection and academic failure. It often took several attempts for him to process incoming information correctly. I couldn't wait to get to the car to share the good news with him once more.

"Cognitive neurologist" was a new term for me. The specialist practiced at a major teaching hospital about an hour's drive from home and, with the local neurologist's help, we were able to secure an appointment for the following week. On the day of the appointment, Luke's demeanor was more relaxed than it had been in some time, and he actually smiled at me during breakfast and asked when we were leaving. I wondered if these small shifts in attitude and posture indicated that he sensed his life was about to change for the better. He was obviously willing to take another try at help, and I wondered if he knew that this appointment held more promise than usual, coming on the heels of a diagnosis that finally made full sense. Since Luke had no memory of life before injury, it would be difficult for him to comprehend what his life could be like once he received the targeted help he so badly needed. But, having been mocked and socially rejected, and hearing Mark's and my concerns and those of his teachers voiced on an almost daily basis, he was aware that the life he was living held far more challenges than he could easily handle. In the back of my own mind, doubts lurked; my trust in the medical profession had been sorely eroded over so many years. Pushing the doubts down, I returned Luke's smile, and we headed to the car.

The specialist took Luke's history for almost an hour and a half, although Luke was a passive participant for much of that time. After giving his HIPAA permission for the physician to talk to me, Luke fell asleep in the examining room chair, and the doctor let him sleep. At the end of the ninety minutes, he said to me, "I'm going to order a scan of Luke's brain." That had never been done before. An element of renewed hope jumped uninvited into my thoughts. Maybe these two new doctors really were in our corner and on the right track, but I wasn't ready yet to cast aside all doubt.

He then declared, in no uncertain terms, that Luke's difficulties resulted from a traumatic brain injury, or TBI, caused by the blow to his head at the playground so many years earlier. He believed it was a mild injury and that the SPECT scan, a nuclear imaging test that would produce a three-dimensional picture of Luke's brain, would come back negative as, he explained, they often do in the case of mild brain injuries.

"But don't think for a moment that this is not a brain injury," he announced. His words etched themselves into my own brain. He expressed concern and confusion that this injury had remained undiagnosed for so many years, explaining that the disparity between Luke's high IQ and his failure to succeed academically was a hallmark of TBI, and that the school system should have picked up the divergence years earlier. "I don't know how this was missed," he said sadly.

At that point, I still had no clear understanding of the clinical implications of brain injury. The term "traumatic brain injury" was new to me, and, although I had all along believed Luke had sustained some kind of injury to his head or brain from the accident with the swing, I had no idea what that meant medically. I was, to say the least, overwhelmed by all the information the doctor was providing.

I asked about the ADHD diagnosis Luke had been given and if that diagnosis still applied. He explained that Luke's ADHD classification likely arose from the TBI and was just one of the overt manifestations of the injury itself. Since Luke's short trial run on the ADHD medication several years earlier had not produced helpful results, the neurologist didn't suggest trying it again at this point. "Let's wait to see what the scan shows, and we'll proceed from there."

For several days after the appointment, the sensation of sudden clarity had me walking with my feet off the ground. After all those years of confusion, this revelation changed absolutely everything. I found it amazing and unsettling all at once.

With all of the previously unanswered questions about Luke now incorporated within this overarching diagnosis, the gate to so many more questions was thrown wide open. How would the diagnosis of traumatic brain injury affect Luke's future? I naively assumed it would bring with it options and a cure. How would the injury be repaired? Would Luke need to have surgery? Would that be dangerous, and how long would the recovery be?

Yet the unknown implications running as new questions through my brain were held at bay by an odd sense of joy. For the first time in sixteen years, hope that Luke would now have the opportunity to live a happy, productive life seemed bolstered by reality. I felt giddy; I felt like dancing. In fact, I felt so happy I could hardly sleep during the next several days. Through it all, my energy levels held, and life seemed good for the first time in a very long time.

Mark and Luke, however, were more reserved. "Let's wait for the scan results," Mark had said when I described my infusion of hope after the visit to the doctor, and he quickly went back to reading his book. A portion of his less-than-ebullient response was due to so many years of disappointment. That was obvious. His personal methodology, however, played a larger role in his wait-and-see response. Mark is a thorough thinker, and he doesn't react quickly. My marked enthusiasm was no doubt a tad annoying to him, but he never let on, nor did he say a word to discourage me.

Luke maintained his flat expression after the diagnosis was pronounced, and yet he seemed more emotionally available than he had been in quite a while. He quietly chuckled at my expressions of joy, and willingly played card games with me for the first time in years. Of course, only the diagnosis had been made; there had not yet been any treatment. Luke was no more capable of reading quickly and accurately or of processing information correctly than he had been prior to the diagnosis. We had yet to discover what treatment for Luke would entail, and, as I looked at him studying his cards, I couldn't help but wonder what the next few weeks would bring. I was certain that once family and friends learned about this definitive TBI diagnosis, they would begin to show more support and encouragement.

The scan was scheduled for the following week. The test required an intravenous injection in Luke's arm with a radioactive dye, and then an hour-long wait before the scan was performed. Luke and I passed the time eating lunch on a park bench outside the hospital cafeteria. I sensed his agitation and anticipation, and it dawned on me that during the past few days he had perhaps begun to process all this new information about having a brain injury. *What was going through his head? Was he fearful of the unknown, in terms of treatment and repair? Did he realize the relief that this diagnosis could bring to his life? Did the fact that Luke's injury was to his brain imply that he might not fully process what was happening?* As we stood up and walked toward the radiology lab, Luke caught my eye for a moment. He didn't say a word, but the set of his face was determined. I returned his glance with a smile and a nod of my head, which I hope he understood. I believe Luke and I both at that moment recognized the importance of what he was about to do, and that, for the first time since the accident, help might be just a test away. I reminded myself that the doctor had warned us that the results would likely come back as normal since mild TBI often doesn't show on a scan. But internally, I was counting on it showing us something that could help Luke. I knew from past experiences that hard evidence might be the only way to dispel doubt and lead to viable treatment options.

I tried to put my arm through Luke's, but he pulled away. I retreated and was grateful he had at least made eye contact with me in a meaningful way. Ever since his freshman year of high school, Luke seemed to take on the world in sparring mode, and I prayed at that moment that one of the benefits of this diagnosis might be a renewed trust in people. As I watched Luke follow the technicians into the testing area, I also prayed that as he matured, he might accept a hug once in awhile and allow some of his lurking anger and fear to melt away. Luke often reminded me of a flailing, drowning swimmer, fighting off the very help he desperately needed.

The two-week wait for the follow-up neurology appointment seemed endless. Surely, no matter what the scan showed, the diagnosis of traumatic brain injury resulting from his playground accident sixteen years earlier would stand and would lead to help for Luke. The doctor had been insistent about that, and it was the only logical explanation for Luke's experiences.

Mark joined us for the scheduled return visit, and I couldn't wait for him to hear the diagnosis directly from the doctor's lips. I had shared with him what we had learned, but there is nothing as powerful as hearing the words firsthand. This was finally an opportunity to bridge the emotional rifts that had developed in our family during the years that Luke's injury remained unidentified.

I had confidence in our family's future as we sat in the waiting room. I closed my eyes and daydreamed about how Mark and I would finally learn how to help Luke; and how Luke, more importantly, would have a clearly defined path toward a happily productive life.

And then, returning to reality somewhat, my thoughts leveled and accepted that, without clear-cut, definitive evidence of injury on the scan, help for Luke might only be another pipe dream. Fortunately, just as my apprehension darkened, the doctor came through the door and handed us news that altered the course of all of our lives.

"Luke's brain scan was positive," he began. "I wasn't expecting this. This is not just a mild injury, and I don't know how he has made it as far as he has all these years."

But Mark and I both knew. Since middle school, we had helped Luke every step of the way, because his failures wouldn't have been learning opportunities—they would have buried him. The realization of our enabling was very uncomfortable, as it had been at every turn. We wished for healthy independence for Luke, independence with a solid foundation of self-assurance and self-reliance. Realizing we were continuing to enable him was exactly what had made us so uneasy as Luke grew older while his skill levels remained stagnant at increasingly low levels relative to his advancing age. Now it seemed the source of Luke's mounting failures and of our confusion and worry was suddenly right in front of us, pictured on the brain scan.

I watched as the doctor pointed to the area of injury on the scan, and I trembled. Even with no medical background, I could easily see where the flow of blood narrowed considerably, corresponding to the part of Luke's brain that had been struck by the swing. The injury was visibly outlined, even to my untrained eye. My pulse quickened with the painful but clear realization that there it was, proof positive that Luke had actually sustained the injury I had suspected for so long.

"So, what do we do now, Doctor?" I asked, snapping out of the shock and eager to get to the task of "curing" Luke. "Where do we go from here? What's the next step?" I was anticipating a litany of choices—options that would help our son find his way back to the normalcy that we all so desperately wanted.

Instead, the abruptness of the doctor's answer jarred me from my thoughts of help and hope. I will never forget his words.

"Oh, there's nothing to do. Your son's life is over. It is way too late for him."

A Bird in the Hand

The shock and insensitivity of the doctor's words made me lightheaded. I struggled to breathe normally.

"That can't be true! Surely there's something you can do for Luke. We can't have waited this long for his injury to be identified, just to be told now that there's nothing to be done for our son. That can't be!"

The doctor gave a little smile that I couldn't interpret. He stood and began walking to the door. Mark and Luke stood and followed him, but I couldn't immediately get my bearings.

"I'm sorry," he said, having now opened the door into the waiting area. I stood up and wiped away my tears as we exited. The door closed behind us. This was the one outcome I had not even considered.

I did not believe the doctor; I *could not* believe him. How could we have reached this point of finally having hard-copy diagnostic evidence of the source of Luke's problems, only to be told there was nothing we could do to help him? I simply could not accept that answer. If this doctor wouldn't help us, surely someone else would.

Once home, I picked up the phone and began calling Luke's tutors, looking for any suggestions they might have in light of the now-definitive TBI diagnosis. I still didn't understand what having a brain injury implied, even in the simplest of terms. I had never known anyone with a brain injury, and the only picture of TBI I had in my own mind had little to do with Luke's manifestations. Luke was not in a wheelchair; he walked and talked normally. My preconceptions clearly needed adjusting.

One of the tutors had a lead: he told me about a neuropsychologist with whom he had worked, years earlier. The most recent information he had was that his former coworker ran a program, commutable from where we lived, to rehabilitate people with brain injuries. I was able to locate the neuropsychologist's contact number, and to my surprise, I reached him immediately. He told me his program for people with traumatic brain injuries was still in operation, and we proceeded to have a lively and interesting conversation. I provided the quick version, basic highlights of the past sixteen years, and then it was his turn.

"Let me tell you about your son," he said. And, with startling clarity, he did. He described the sudden change of behavior and personality after the swing accident, including the anxiety and agitation that had immediately resulted. He described Luke's inability to succeed, which didn't become overtly apparent until middle school. He described Luke's social difficulties and his inability to focus in team settings, whether for sports or school projects. Then he spoke aloud the pieces of the puzzle that were the most frightening to Mark and me: the out-of-control teenage behavior with increasing levels of impulsivity, defiance, disrespect, poor judgment, acting out, and sudden raging anger against us.

He went on to give Luke a voice that rang intensely true. He said that Luke thought of himself as worthless since, without a diagnosis for so many years, he had only himself to blame for his failures. He told me it was logical that Luke's sense of failure and the fear and frustration that accompanied it would result in the anger he directed at Mark and me. Because Luke had watched Mark and me succeed, he expected to follow suit, and when he failed, he felt all the worse about himself. The doctor explained that although I described Luke's natural personality as sweet, docile, and kind, the injury to his brain made it impossible for him to achieve his goals, increasing his frustration and self-doubt. Frustration and doubt were then filtered through a damaged brain, which was unable to process information correctly to produce a reasonable response to his negative emotions.

I mentioned Luke's description of the five televisions all going at once without an "off" switch. The neuropsychologist wasn't surprised, and even expressed sympathy for the burden Luke carried with him unceasingly, day in and day out. When I told him that smoking pot was the only thing that quieted those noises for Luke, he accepted this without judgment. He explained that, in an attempt to salve his presumption of worthlessness and to quiet those relentless noises within his brain, Luke had learned to self-medicate with marijuana. He also told me that Luke was not alone among those with TBI in making that choice.

Before our conversation ended, the director invited Mark and me to visit the program before mentioning it to Luke. Then his voice took a serious tone: "Luke has suffered too many failures already, and he cannot suffer another major failure here." He didn't spell out in words what that next failure would do to our son, but his meaning was clear. Luke simply could not and would not recover from it.

Despite that dire warning, I found truth and encouragement in his words, so Mark and I made an appointment to meet with him and his staff the following Monday morning, by now well into April. While there, we also met nine or ten people who were participating in the brain injury treatment program, as well as the family member or friend accompanying each, as the program required. We spent time observing the interactions between the ten participants and the staff, and tried to picture Luke there. All of the participants were older than Luke, but a few, at least, were somewhat close to his age. We knew nothing about the field of brain injury rehabilitation, but we found the approximate two-to-one ratio between participants and staff an encouraging sign. The program director had an impressive professional pedigree, and the program was backed by a major large-city hospital. The director and staff did not provide us with any reason during our observation why their program couldn't or wouldn't work for our son. The assumption that the plan *might* work, however, came with a caveat. The staff forewarned us that the long delay in Luke's diagnosis had led to well-entrenched dysfunction, and they could offer no guarantee of success.

I shuddered, recalling the neuropsychologist's warning: *Luke has suffered too many failures already . . .* How were we to assess what we had just witnessed? Our visit that morning consisted of sitting in with the group of learners and their family members, all in one room, with one person receiving attention and feedback as the designated member of the day. The staff discussed with her the plan of action they had previously assigned to her, and then evaluated her progress with it. The other participants also gave feedback and encouragement, one by one, as did the family members of all participants. We saw no one-to-one remediation efforts, and were told those took place in the afternoons. In many ways, I felt as though we were watching a foreign movie without subtitles. The TBI terms used so freely in the discussions were not words Mark and I understood well. By noon, when we said our goodbyes, I felt lost and confused.

Over a quick lunch, Mark and I realized we had no way to determine if this program would work for Luke. We were untrained, and would have to simply trust that this option was a viable one. Although there were apparently other programs in the city for TBI rehabilitation, we knew of none specifically, and we both agreed that this "bird in the hand" seemed like a reasonable plan of action. It certainly had a stellar reputation, and the staff had voted to accept Luke if he was willing to attend. We decided to tell Luke about it and go from there.

When we described the program to Luke, his face lit up and he stood a bit straighter than he had in quite a while. Mornings were perpetually difficult for Luke, but he managed to be ready on time to make the hour-and-forty-minute journey to the program center for the first of four days of scheduled midmorning neuropsychological testing. That first day of testing exhausted him, but the next day he cooperated sufficiently to catch the train into the city with me with a few minutes to spare. By the third day, rousing Luke was more difficult, and on the fourth day it presented quite a challenge. And yet, once up and dressed, he seemed anxious to get into the city and get the testing underway. Exhausted as he was, he clearly wanted the help this program might offer.

Luke's test results revealed specific traumatic brain injury impairments; and, center stage in a room filled with the other TBI participants, their attending family members, the staff, director, and co-director, he was offered the opportunity to return in the fall to begin treatment. Mark and I had previously described the program to him as a "thirteenth year" of study, a concept familiar to him from his stay at the boarding school. Luke still held hope of becoming a physicist and wanted to attend college, and he knew this program could be his chance to follow that dream.

Without hesitating, Luke nodded his acceptance. He also flashed his oh-so-endearing smile that manifested a sense of accomplishment, so we knew even he had found reason to hope.

But first Luke had to figure out how to graduate high school.

A Push to Graduation

As soon as we had the definitive brain injury diagnosis in hand, we called for another appointment with the school's child study team. The educational advocate had informed us that, due to the diagnosis, the school district was obligated to continue Luke's education to the age of twenty-one, if we wanted that extension. Since that would preclude him from graduating with his class, we felt Luke should be involved in making the decision. He was adamant that all he wanted was to graduate on time and with his friends. Still, Mark and I wanted to find out what the school's child study team might offer once they learned of Luke's newly defined diagnosis, so we went ahead with the meeting.

The moment we uttered the words "traumatic brain injury," the members of the team shared furtive glances, not lost on us. They promptly interrupted the conversation and withdrew for a team conference.

If they had waited, they would have heard us say that, although he was entitled to continued assistance for several more years at state expense, Luke wanted only to graduate with his class. He had begged Mark and me for that opportunity, and we had decided Luke's self-esteem was more valuable than any state program for continuing education might be.

Instead, when the team returned a few minutes later, they stated firmly that Luke was to be put on home study immediately, but that he would graduate with his class. No one mentioned the option of keeping him in the system for the next several years. Although I was pleased that Luke's wish to graduate with his class would be granted (in spite of failing grades in virtually every class), I was appalled that this group of professionals would by omission deny parents the opportunity to make an informed decision. If the advocate had never mentioned the state regulation permitting Luke to continue school to age twenty-one, we would never have known the option existed.

Luke's high school days were immediately over. A tutor arranged by the school came to our home for several hours every weekday for the next several months until graduation, but if educational achievement was the goal, it was lost on me. Whatever schoolwork they accomplished was minimal at best, but Luke seemed to enjoy the arrangement. No doubt he missed seeing his friends, but he liked having most of the day available for video games and sleeping.

I hated the setup, but I bit my tongue and let it play out. Luke would graduate with his friends, and I desperately hoped he would be able to patch the holes in his educational mortar once his brain injury was treated. I couldn't wait for September to arrive.

We had no idea what the future held for Luke, but we wanted to provide him with a sense of attainment, even if it were largely an empty one. For Luke, however, that diploma was a symbol of hope. He believed the remediation he would receive at the brain injury rehabilitation facility would solve his cognitive problems and that he could then become a physicist. The diploma embodied all his dreams for success at that moment, and neither Mark nor I was about to shatter them.

Another Kind of Rehab

The summer between graduation and the start of the brain injury treatment program was extremely challenging for our family, despite the prospects for help that awaited us in the fall.

It was becoming more obvious that Luke was smoking pot regularly. His eyes were clouded and his mood darkened. Despite my naivete about drugs of any kind, I knew drug use was the wrong path for any adolescent, especially one who couldn't grasp the connection between actions and consequences. Instinct told me that if Luke were to fall prey to the lure of drugs and become addicted, that disconnect would preclude him from seeing that drugs were negatively impacting his life, and from realizing he'd have to change his actions to break the addiction.

In light of the TBI diagnosis, Mark and I saw that summer as a fresh start for our son. We believed that with a high school diploma in hand Luke could eventually attend college; but first he had to clean up his act and take a little time in the fall for the brain injury professionals to teach him how to read properly and overcome some of his other academic obstacles. Knowing absolutely nothing about closed-head traumatic brain injury, I assumed that almost all of Luke's academic problems stemmed from his difficulty with reading comprehension and that, because of his high IQ, that deficit could be easily fixed once treatment began. I even wondered whether Luke might "graduate" from the program earlier than the scheduled twenty weeks.

Luke was adamant that he did not want to start college midyear. He had been so conscious of his differences throughout high school that he wanted to begin college in the fall like most other freshmen. Realizing that those few weeks of reading remediation in the fall would cost Luke a full year's delay entering college agitated me. I began pondering what kind of interim job Luke might find between the completion of the brain injury training and the start of the next fall semester, almost a year later. I was having trouble staying "in the moment." By this point, I had forgotten how to relax.

With only a sporadic caddying job to keep him busy, Luke's verbal outbursts increased during those first few weeks after graduation, his frustrations escalating to monstrous proportions. He was closing in on his nineteenth birthday and still had to be nagged and cajoled out of bed every morning. Knowing he would soon be an adult responsible for his own livelihood, and not realizing at the time that his brain injury was likely playing a role in Luke's aversion to work, Mark and I pushed him, and often pushed him hard.

Whenever Mark would press Luke to get out of the house to go to his caddying job, Luke would respond by yelling at his father at the top of his lungs, just like he screamed at me for asking him to help with chores. Neither of us knew what to do or how to fix this beastly living situation, and September felt an eternity away. The tension in our house was so thick it seemed almost visible.

Luke's high school guidance counselor appeared to genuinely care about him, and prior to graduation she had made efforts to come up with a workable summer plan. She gave me a brochure advertising a camp for highly functioning kids with learning disabilities. I looked into it and, following several phone conversations, was left with a favorable impression of the people who ran it. I phoned parents of kids Luke's age who had attended, and received good feedback. Luke, with his usual unenthusiastic demeanor, agreed to participate in the program. It consisted of a two-week trip in the northwestern US and parts of British Columbia, scheduled to begin in just a few weeks. Despite the drain on our finances, it sounded ideal.

Mark and I had become accustomed by this point to the exorbitant expense of raising a child with what turned out to be a brain injury. Our son's life was at stake, and if keeping him on track meant hiring an educational consultant or another tutor or psychologist, it was worth every penny. This time, spending money to give him a couple of weeks with other kids who struggled every day seemed reasonable. But these expenditures came with an element of discomfort; there was no way to determine if the people and programs we invested in would lead to success for our son. It had taken sixteen years just to find a physician knowledgeable enough about TBI to identify it in Luke, and that delay told us that this condition was not well recognized or understood. But we had to do something.

On the day Luke was to leave, Mark and I took him to the airport where he was to meet his traveling companions for the first time. We respected his desire to do the meet-and-greet on his own, but I admit I peeked around pillars to ensure not only that my about-to-be-nineteen-year-old-going-on-twelve found the camp counselors, but also that the group as a whole passed my maternal litmus test. When the counselors reached out to shake Luke's hand and seemed to demonstrate kind consideration to each camper, I breathed a sigh of relief and prayed that Luke would have a good time and form some lasting friendships. It was certainly a highly recommended organization, so I allowed myself to relax and assume all would be fine.

Four days after Luke's departure, Mark and I went away for the weekend. When I turned on my cell phone the first evening to check my messages, I was startled by the number of calls I had missed. They were all from one of the camp counselors, and when I called him back, he seemed overly relieved to hear my voice.

"We are sending Luke home on the next flight," he told me. "Please be at the airport to pick him up." As Mark and I scurried to pack and drive back home, I relayed the phone conversation to him.

Luke had run away from the group while they were in British Columbia and had been gone for nine hours before they found him and convinced him to return to camp.

By law, Luke was an adult and could have refused to return with the counselor. Knowing how impulsive his behavior was and how poorly he processed information, I knew he could have easily run away without realizing the dangers he faced until it was too late. I could barely breathe during the long ride home. I tried hard to mask my fears in front of Mark, but by this point, my body, mind, and soul were riddled with angst, and I failed miserably. I sobbed quietly, then tried to calm myself for a while; but the tears soon returned. Mark insisted on dropping me at home first so I could rest, and then continued the final hour-long stretch to the airport, arriving in the middle of the night just in time to see his fatigued, filthy son disembark from the flight.

The camp counselor had speculated that Luke had likely run away because he'd been caught using a cold medicine in an apparent attempt to get high. He'd also been seen trying to snort some ADHD medication one of the campers had. *Snort ADHD medication? What did that mean? Luke had been prescribed ADHD medication in high school. If it was safe for him to swallow, how would he think snorting it or another medication like it would make him high?* I was so confused and frightened and angry—at Luke and for him.

I fully admit Luke could have benefitted from having a set of parents with more knowledge about drug abuse than either Mark or I had. We knew Luke used marijuana occasionally, although we found it on him only once. And now this. In spite of my cluelessness, I knew substance abuse was not only dangerous for Luke, but was likely exacerbating his behavioral outbursts, so once he was back home and cleaned up, we immediately made arrangements for him to participate in a local drug rehabilitation program. Even though it was outpatient only, it had a good reputation and success record. And he could get started right away.

Mark and I had leveraged options so deeply with our son that we had little clout left, short of permanently canceling his cell phone and kicking him out of the house. His video games had recently been put under lock and key and he no longer had access to our cars. The only thing left that he valued enough to possibly alter his behavior was his cell phone. Under normal circumstances, I would have had no problem canceling that cell phone, but Luke had remained confusingly more like a preteen than a late teen in terms of maturity, and I couldn't bring myself to cut off permanently what I perceived to be his only link to safety. I periodically pored over the itemized phone bills and kept track of the numbers he called and received, and I rationalized that spying on Luke via his cell phone was helping to keep him safe by providing us with a list of his contacts and even his whereabouts.

I had no idea of the full extent of Luke's marijuana use; all I knew was that he thought he needed to "quiet the noises" in his brain. I've often thought back to when he told me about those noises in his head years earlier, and how angry I was with myself for not having found an answer for him at the time. Realizing now that the cacophony of noise had continued unabated for all these years made me feel sick all over. Luke never explicitly told me that drugs also eased his sense of personal failure, but that would certainly make sense. I tried putting myself in his place and was sure that, if I heard noises constantly and had endured failure upon failure without understanding why, I might have turned to drugs also.

The local outpatient drug treatment center wasn't able to help Luke. He acted out in sessions and refused to participate. In addition, he met people whose drug problems far exceeded his own. One day, he brought a young man home with him, and the two of them looked stoned out of their minds. I called Luke into another room, explained that his guest had to leave, and offered to drive him home. At first they agreed, but as soon as we all walked outside toward the car, the two of them ran into the nearby woods, laughing like naughty children. Luke's lagging maturity had always been out of balance with his growing body, but the addition of marijuana worsened everything. Feeling powerless and having no idea what to do next, I sat on the driveway and sobbed.

The only hope now for Luke, in my mind, was an inpatient drug rehabilitation program. We still did not believe Luke was using hard-core drugs, but we were terrified that this would be the next step. It seemed crucial that we stop him before he reached the point of no return. Looking back, I now understand that Luke's behavior was likely driven by his brain injury, and that treating the brain injury first would have been the more targeted approach. At the time, however, I equated keeping him free of drugs with keeping him safe, and I wanted my son to be safe. More than anything, I wanted Luke to be safe.

Through additional networking and research, two options emerged. One was an inpatient drug program about three hours from home that had a high success rate. I explained Luke's recent diagnosis of traumatic brain injury to them, and they assured me they understood the situation. By then, with my own resources spent, I was a quick believer in any positive statement that represented hope. Unfortunately, Luke was ineligible to enter the adolescent program because he had recently turned nineteen, and they would make no exceptions, despite my concerns about Luke's immaturity and about exposing him to addicts who could teach him more than he already knew.

The next option I found was also residential, but it had the added benefit of being a dual-diagnosis program, covering both cognitive help for TBI and substance abuse. One of the directors made the ninety-minute drive to our home and spent a few hours interviewing both Luke and me. He was soft-spoken and kind, and explained that TBI often goes hand in hand with substance abuse, reassuring me that Luke's self-medicating was not unusual. The program sounded ideal to me. Luke, however, preferred waiting for the brain injury rehabilitation program he had visited, thinking that would provide the best chance for him to be able to attend college. So we made the decision to forgo the residential dual-diagnosis option and wait until September for in-depth treatment of his cognitive brain injury deficits. It was the logical choice, but the problem of Luke's growing dependence on marijuana and his increasing verbal outbursts and behavioral misjudgments remained. *How in the world could Luke find success cognitively if substance abuse got in the way?*

I decided to contact the psychologist who had worked with Luke during high school, and who had developed a good relationship with him in the process. Surely he would be able to help guide us through this maze of options. He agreed that the brain injury treatment, scheduled to begin in only a few short months, had far greater potential for success if Luke were clean and sober.

Luke's excitement over the prospect of finding help at the brain injury program in the large nearby city became our carrot. Mark and I talked with him at length about his need to quit using marijuana in order to succeed there. He agreed with us, in theory at least, and we told him about the inpatient drug rehabilitation program we'd found. "Later," he said. We reiterated the importance of starting the brain injury program in the fall with a clear head. He seemed to understand and to agree that time was short to accomplish that goal, since it was already early August.

The following week, the three of us took a short vacation, but before we left, Mark and I made arrangements to drop Luke off at the inpatient drug-only rehab program on the way home, and we verbalized those plans to Luke. As we ended our vacation, we had another talk with Luke about the benefits of the program and again voiced our plan to enroll him at the center the following day. To our surprise, Luke appeared to have come to grips with his need for sobriety, and to understand its importance prior to the start of the TBI program in the fall. We were delighted by his acquiescence.

When we arrived at the rehab facility, however, it became clear that Luke had processed our conversations completely differently than we had. He'd apparently not realized he was being asked to immediately enter a drug treatment program, and had somehow assumed in spite of our conversations to the contrary that when he did participate sometime in the unspecified future, it would be a stay of only a day or two at most. Standing in the lobby of the rehab building, he suddenly realized what was happening and flew into an impetuous rage. His face was the picture of fear. In spite of attempts by the professionals to calm him, Luke bolted from one entrance hallway to the next before barging out the door and running down the steps to our car.

What happened next was unbelievable to me. Our precious son pulled a cigarette lighter from his pocket and opened the cap on the car's gas tank. With body and hands shaking, he yelled that he would ignite the tank and blow himself up. I was so scared, the only thing I could do was call out to him, over and over again. "Luke, don't! Luke! Luke, get away from the car!" The administrators forced me into a room where I couldn't see what was happening. I heard sirens and, as they drew closer, I realized I didn't know if Luke was alive or dead. I didn't think I'd heard an explosion, but I wondered if I could be wrong. Fortunately, when the police arrived, they recognized that Luke's actions stemmed from fear, and within moments of their arrival, the crisis came to an end. The police told Luke they would not arrest him, and the facility would not press charges, but only if he agreed to check himself into rehab. Frightened by the intensity of his own actions, Luke agreed.

Mark accompanied him into a small administrative office to complete the paperwork. I began to doubt our decision to leave Luke there, given his obvious fear and the threat of suicide, but I realized we could not back down. Rewarding Luke's aggressive behavior would only make matters worse. Luke was in good hands, and we put our fragile faith in that. *Who better to help him?* Certainly not Mark and I, since neither of us had any kind of psychological or drug abuse training. Luke desperately needed professional help. *Was this the best way to provide it for him?* There were no clear-cut answers, and that was unsettling, but as Mark and I walked out of the building and headed toward the car, numbness took over.

The emotional toll of Luke's long-undiagnosed TBI had nearly broken our family. The pain of watching our son endure failure upon failure and slide into visible signs of depression and helplessness and self-medication was crippling to Mark and me. We loved our child beyond reason, but we had become the target for his expressions of pain—verbal outbursts that could only be categorized as abusive. That abuse, combined with the lack of a sense of emotional connection with Luke, was horrendously painful. Traumatic brain injury is indeed a family illness, and a devastating condition.

My anxiety about leaving Luke at the inpatient program seemed illogically at odds with the emotional release I felt as we drove away that day. The escalation of Luke's verbally abusive outbursts had become overwhelming, and neither Mark nor I could predict whether our son would be lion or lamb on any given day. The lamb days, when Luke remained calm and sweet-natured, were becoming fewer and farther between. On the days when the lion roared, he often shouted obscenities at us, always without making direct eye contact. It was as though he was looking past us as he bellowed, and his bellowing never quite matched the circumstances. When he yelled at the space around us instead of directly at us, it often seemed he just needed to vent, and we happened to be handy. Yes, he was angry; and yes, the anger was a clear expression of frustration, but none of it made sense. I had learned to walk on eggshells and had grown exhausted in the process. Mark and I were both emotionally depleted and badly in need of some respite away from Luke, so that we could re-energize and refocus our attention on meeting his escalating needs. Secondarily, we hoped Luke's time away from home might break the untenable behavioral patterns that had been consuming all of us.

On the ride home, I thought back to an incident from the previous year, when one of our former neighbors had visited. We had taken a long walk, and she asked how Luke was doing. Still almost a year away from diagnosis, Luke was knee-deep in failure.

"He's not doing very well. He's having difficulty finding success and is becoming quite a handful."

The neighbor suggested that since "the apple doesn't fall far from the tree," I should step in and get to work with Luke—blatantly implying that his failures were a direct consequence of poor parenting. Her words stung deeply. Now, a year later, it was obvious that the parenting tactics we had applied had been wholly ineffective, and we had to trust that removing Luke from drugs through inpatient rehabilitation and allowing time for rest and rejuvenation for all of us would be the answer.

Just when we needed it most, though, relaxation was yanked from us by yet another crisis. Our lives and our anticipation of good things to come were once again upended.

On the third day of Luke's rehabilitation, we received an unexpected call. Luke had run away from the facility the previous day. A member of the staff had followed him, and he had finally agreed to return to the center, after many hours of what was described as "disconnected conversation." I'd barely survived the camp escapade earlier that summer and Luke's two disappearances the previous year, and I didn't know how much more my mind and body could tolerate.

The rehab counselor asked me a lot of questions about the traumatic brain injury diagnosis, which they had initially told me they understood relative to addiction treatment. The counselor then assured me they would be able to help Luke and that a treatment breakthrough usually occurs within the first several days, so Luke's should come soon. There had never been a quick fix for Luke before, but, knowing little to nothing about drug rehabilitation, I trusted that he would fall into the category of what "usually" happened.

Instead, the next day, I received an even more terrifying phone call. By now, my body went on high alert every time the phone rang when Luke was out of the house, but I still wasn't prepared for this call. This time, Luke had become so behaviorally impulsive and verbally abusive that the counselors had made the decision to remove him from the program. Several hours earlier, he had been handed his duffel bag and his cell phone and was asked to leave. In Luke's case, they said, there was something very wrong with his mental processing, and they strongly encouraged us to get to him as quickly as we could and take him home. They told us Luke needed help and needed it now. With that, the conversation ended as abruptly as it had begun.

We knew Luke had left the rehab building, located in a rural, wooded area a three-hour drive from our home, but we didn't know where he'd gone after that. It was already almost four in the afternoon. I phoned Mark at work. Darkness would set in before we could get to Luke, and we decided having both of us there to search for him if necessary was better than one of us going alone. When Mark arrived home a very long hour later, we quickly set out for the grueling ride ahead. Mercifully, an hour into the trip, we were finally able to reach Luke by cell phone, and we arranged a meeting place. Still, there was no way of knowing if he would actually be there. My heart was beating out of my chest by the time we rounded the last corner before our destination and saw Luke sitting on the side of the road. He yelled and cursed at us the whole way home, but I found comfort in simply having him with us, safe and sound.

I made an appointment to speak again with Luke's psychologist the following week to try to form some new plan of action. Fortunately, I was allowed continued access to Luke's information since Luke had signed a HIPAA confidentiality waiver when he began treatment. The counselor now felt it would be unwise to take further action relative to drug abuse at this point, and advised that we pin our hope for guidance on the TBI treatment program closer to home that fall.

Mark and I concurred. We didn't know what else to do.

Finally, September

So we set our sights and hopes on September and began to think about the logistics of the three of us commuting over an hour each way into the city. Each TBI program participant was required to have a relative or caregiver attend the program also, and I looked forward to that assignment, if not the commute. I knew the Monday-through-Thursday travel would sap Luke's energy, since fatigue was ever-present for him. And when he became fatigued, he acted out. I worried exhaustion would interfere with his ability to absorb the treatment.

In the end, Mark, who had endured a long commute for many years, made the decision. Rather than all of us spending long hours in transit, he suggested it might be better to rent an apartment in the city. With a short window of time before the program was to begin, we put our house on the market. If the house sold, we would make the move into the city; if not, the three of us would tackle the rails.

Three days later, we were in the midst of a bidding war on our house—one decision made easy. We had planned to build a home for retirement in another state in a year or two anyway, and now that this house was sold, we could use our time in the city to plan for that dream. I spent a day apartment shopping there with a friend, but I couldn't picture us in any of the four or five modern units we saw. As time with the real estate agent was winding down, I asked if there was anything available in an older, more solid building. Underlying my doubts about the other units were their thinner walls and my fear that, if Luke's verbal outbursts continued unabated, we might risk eviction. In her last fifteen minutes of available time, the agent showed us a unit that finally felt like home, thick walls included. The next day, Mark took a look and signed the rental agreement.

We moved in on a Friday, just in time to settle into apartment living before beginning the brain injury treatment program the following Monday. Luke had dealt with the move to the city with as much passivity as he seemed capable of mustering at that point, and on our first evening there, he chose to stay in the apartment while Mark and I ventured out for dinner. We weren't gone long, so when we returned, we were surprised to find Luke already asleep in his new room. The next day, he played video games and slept, but he did rally enough to go out with us for an evening walk. By the end of the weekend, Luke seemed a little more at ease in his surroundings, and I hoped he wouldn't get antsy and impulsively go out in search of anything troublesome. I worried about the new forms of danger that might await him in this large city.

On Monday morning, Luke and I set out in plenty of time to make the mile-and-a-half journey to the TBI program. On the bus, it was obvious Luke wanted to ride in silence, so I had twenty minutes to ponder how the day would go and to try to calm my nervous enthusiasm. In my ignorance about traumatic brain injury, I expected Luke would be the most highly functioning person in the program, requiring only some strategic skills to improve his reading comprehension. I still believed remediation would be completed quickly.

I soon learned how mistaken I was. That first morning after introductions, the participants shared their personal stories; by lunchtime, I felt overwhelmed and already exhausted. With the exception of one person whose TBI affected his ability to speak, if I had met any of these participants anywhere but here, I wouldn't have realized any of them had a brain injury.

They had all sustained relatively recent injuries that had required some degree of hospitalization, and those with the more severe injuries had been sent from the hospital to specialized medical rehabilitation centers to address their semi-acute needs, such as walking, talking, and relearning basic personal care skills. Having accomplished all of that over months of time, they were now ready to tackle remediation for their cognitive deficits. Like so many others who are uninformed, I had erroneously assumed that once an injured brain had relearned the basics, the rest would just fall into place.

Because Luke had never been hospitalized and had remained undiagnosed for the first sixteen years after injury, his situation was quite different from that of the others enrolled in this program. He had no prior knowledge of how his injury had affected his life, nor any memory of life before injury, and he had received no help along the way. During the first week of treatment, Luke looked up at the charts of brain injury deficits that hung on every wall and, with sadness in his voice, blurted out, "I have every one of those."

As difficult as it was to accept, I had to agree with him. We were beginning to learn that every facet of Luke's life had been affected, causing his slow start with sociability, his impulsive behaviors, his often-overwhelming fatigue, his reading challenges, his language-processing difficulties that resulted in apples-to-oranges conversations or misconceptions, his quick and angry unfiltered outbursts, the childhood fist-shaking episodes (which we learned were actually seizures), his difficulty modulating his voice at times, and even his malfunctioning body-temperature regulator, which made him feel cold even on very warm days.

Any misconceptions I had that Luke's recovery would be rapid were corrected in short order. Only if Luke were lucky and the stars aligned in his favor would he be able to enter college the following September.

That sudden recognition of how impaired Luke actually was led to several more realizations. First, with each unveiling of an injury deficit that applied to Luke, his previous life experiences, which had made no sense at the time, now made perfect sense. Second, we discovered that this rehabilitation would require more time than any of us had imagined.

Forging new pathways to connect the brain's synapses could be a quite lengthy process, we learned. It dawned on me that it might actually take more than a year for Luke to learn a workable path around his injury to a functional life, and much more time than that to undo the psychological damage that had resulted from being undiagnosed for sixteen years. Finally, little by little, I absorbed the knowledge that success for Luke might not mean a PhD in physics, but might rather mean accepting himself and his limitations, along with a path toward a vocation better suited to both his strengths and weaknesses.

Two things were made very clear to the participants and their family members and caregivers. First, no one's brain injury was going to be "cured"; this was a lifelong disability. But there was hope that, with a lot of hard work, the participants could adopt strategies that would circumvent the injured areas of the brain, and therefore through repetition forge new neural pathways, enabling the individuals to live functional, fulfilling lives. Pre-enrollment testing and staff analysis informed each participant of his or her specific areas of cognitive deficit. Luke's traumatic brain injury had caused difficulty with what they termed "executive functioning" such as planning, organizing, self-modulation, impulse control, and behavioral self-control. Malfunctioning in terms of impulsivity and behavioral outbursts was termed "disinhibition," and the staff chose disinhibition as the initial area of treatment focus for Luke. I had been so honed in on Luke's reading difficulties that this choice startled me, although in retrospect, it made perfect sense to start there. Their logic fit with our growing concerns about Luke's behavioral choices. How could the brain create reconnections if behavioral impulsivity and drug use got in the way?

The idea that Luke's injury wouldn't be cured came as a huge disappointment, but the second point the specialists made really hit home. They stated that brain injury is a family condition, affecting not only the injured person, but every member of the family. All those years of confusion and angst over his academic and social struggles had unquestionably hurt Luke, but Mark's and my anger and hurt at our son's behavioral outbursts had also eroded our own sense of well-being—individually, as a married couple, and as parents. Our ability to blend as a family, to have fun and feel relaxed, had been strained and compromised all those years. This enlightenment was freeing from one perspective, but it also made me want to break down in tears for all the lost time and, most of all, for all of Luke's missed opportunities.

In the late afternoon, when the program let out, Luke would return to the apartment exhausted. He used his energies trying to stay focused during the day, which told me his desire to succeed was strong. Fatigue, I was learning, was the one deficit everyone with a brain injury experiences to varying degrees. That bit of information caused me to reflect on Luke's life experiences and helped to explain why, as a child, he had sometimes put himself to bed in the middle of the day, and why he fell asleep so easily and often. One question answered; so many others yet to comprehend.

The family members and caregivers in the rehabilitation program were encouraged to be a support system for one another, and over lunch we often shared stories of our experiences. Injured at such a young age and undiagnosed for so long afterward, Luke's story was different from those of the other participants, all but one of whom had been injured as adults. Because Luke's injury had remained unidentified for sixteen years, some of the people in that lunchroom couldn't quite relate to our situation. One of the other moms actually told me I had let Luke down by not trying harder. She insisted that her daughter had been diagnosed in less than two years because she had worked tirelessly on her daughter's behalf. So why, she wanted to know, hadn't Luke been diagnosed much earlier, if I had really done my best, as I claimed?

Maybe another parent would have pushed harder for a diagnosis. Maybe I was a lousy, ineffective parent, given Luke's worsening behaviors. Maybe I had failed Luke. My efforts certainly hadn't yielded the results I'd hoped for. And yet, as I look back on it, I know I tried as hard as I knew how. That woman in the lunchroom had dealt with circumstances different from Luke's. Her daughter's benign brain tumor eventually grew large enough to ensure diagnosis. But in Luke's case, until the third neurologist finally ordered a brain scan, Luke's problems had looked like a collection of many other common behavioral or psychological issues, ranging from ADHD to oppositional-defiance disorder to Asperger's syndrome to simple teenage rebellion.

In that moment, however, I left the lunchroom, headed for the hallway, and began to cry. How could one mother who had dealt with so much worry and angst herself turn against another so easily, especially when the circumstances of our children's experiences were so different? Her words crushed me, since of course all I had ever wanted to do was teach my beautiful boy skill sets that would help jumpstart him to his own contented, successful life. Every day in this program I was confronted with the knowledge that my best had not been nearly good enough, and the last thing I needed was another parent casting judgment on top of my own sense of failure.

The program codirector, witnessing my tears, pulled me into her office, where I related the conversation. She explained that even those affected by TBI do not necessarily understand how diagnosis can be a difficult and arduous process. Luke's closed-head injury, although a common variety of TBI, wasn't easily recognizable as it lacked an open wound and because kids often experience head bumps that don't result in brain injury. She drilled home the importance of raising awareness about TBI among physicians, psychologists, teachers, family members, friends, and even those directly dealing with it, so that what happened to Luke wouldn't happen to others. I left her office feeling better, but to this day, frustration at times overwhelms me. *Why should what is unseen be more easily dismissed?* The brain is obviously an essential human organ. Its health directs not just our physical lives, but our behaviors and social interactions. I accept that understanding the workings of the brain is infinitely more difficult than understanding the functions of the liver or kidneys. But I continue to hope that, as research into understanding the brain expands, judgment is reserved and open minds prevail when a person like Luke demonstrates off-the-grid behaviors after having sustained a blow to the head.

Initially, I was so absorbed in the process of learning about TBI and establishing relationships with the other program participants that the fact that we had drawn funds from our dwindling reserves to pay for this expensive program was quickly forgotten. I was so anxious to see Luke restored to full health that it was worth risking financial ruin. But prior to entering the program that September, I had contacted our medical insurance carrier, hoping to allay some of the cost of treatment. The program had dealt with this particular insurance company for many years, and had never once been granted payment from them. So, logically, the program directors fully expected denial of benefits in Luke's case, and they accepted him under the "self-pay" mode. This meant Mark and I were required to pay full program charges up front—which were apparently more than what participating insurance carriers agreed to pay. We had no idea about the financial arrangements of others in the program, but soon learned that most of them were covered by participating medical insurers and/or workmen's compensation. Despite the previous denials, Mark and I made the decision to at least submit the charges to our carrier.

While our insurance company was in the process of reviewing our application, a friend suggested I contact the carrier to request a case manager. When I described Luke's story to the woman assigned to us, she empathically promised she would secure payment for Luke for at least the first twenty-week session. "I won't give up on this," she said, and I believed her. But because this particular insurance company had never approved benefits for this program in the past, I doubted if even this woman's dedication and kindness could overturn such a long history of denials.

Surprisingly, several weeks into the program, we were astonished and grateful to learn that, true to her word, our case manager had indeed secured payment for Luke for the first twenty weeks of treatment. Needless to say, Mark and I were greatly relieved. The expense of moving into the city and renting an apartment was bank-breaking enough. Being spared the burden of also paying out of pocket for the costly TBI treatment was a godsend. It was certainly a day to count our blessings.

Two by the Wayside

I've come to accept that the effects of brain injury are difficult to recognize even when the injury is diagnosed. They can be misunderstood and dismissed, even by professionals, and are all too often disbelieved. Social isolation is apparently a common side effect, as it was for Luke and for me. During the years that Luke's injury remained undiagnosed, and as his academic and social failures increased, friendships were strained by sidelong glances and blunt remarks referencing him or my presumed ineptitude in raising him. For me, feelings of isolation and loneliness became uncomfortable bedfellows to my primary worry about my son. Realizing that Luke was experiencing those same social difficulties as a child made the situation almost unbearable.

Our old neighbor, the one who had made the painful comment about the apple never falling far from the tree, insisted on coming into the city to meet me for lunch once she learned of the TBI diagnosis. I had no desire to see her. I didn't like the way her judgmental tone had made me feel a year earlier and I didn't want to experience more of it. Still, she was persistent, and I allowed hope that with her new knowledge of the diagnosis, we might get back on track. She brought another friend whom I had also known for many years, and the lunch began pleasantly enough. In fact, it felt great at first to reconnect with people I had known for a long time, and in that moment it was easy enough to let go of the hurtful but misinformed comment from the year before. I found my friend's interest in learning about Luke's TBI a positive, welcoming sign.

Once seated at the restaurant, she began asking me about Luke and about the program we were attending. In the midst of relating what I had learned so far and answering her queries, I noticed the unmistakable glances she was directing toward our mutual friend—her raised eyebrows, rolling eyes, and smug smile, as if what I was saying was ludicrous. She had pushed for this meeting, and it suddenly seemed her only motivation was to discount my "excuses" for Luke's poor behavior and failure to succeed. Her disbelief and judgment were palpable and painful to witness, and after about fifteen minutes, I made my excuses, paid for my uneaten lunch, and practically ran from the restaurant.

These were people Mark, Luke, and I had known well and had once counted as friends. Beyond my hurt at their disbelief of Luke's injury and their mockery of him, there was confusion. How could these friends ask about brain injury, share in what I was learning about TBI, and still not believe? I could understand being incredulous that something was physiologically wrong with Luke prior to the diagnosis, but now there were scans and tests to prove it. Why did these people—these friends— cling to their skepticism?

Other friendships, though few, have endured and deepened through it all, and I am grateful for them. Those friends were all the more important and appreciated when others, like the two in the restaurant, denied Luke's injury and offered neither support nor encouragement during our darkest days.

"Hanging by a Thread"

Several weeks into the program, Luke came back to the apartment with me and then announced he was going out for a few minutes. "Okay," I said casually, assuming that, much to my chagrin, he was headed outside for a cigarette. Luke had begun smoking years earlier; it was an addiction that, although harmful to his long-term health, was not a battle I chose to fight at that point.

When he hadn't returned in an hour, I became alarmed and called his cell phone. He didn't answer. I tried again in another half hour. He still didn't answer. I sent him a text message: "Come on in, Luke, supper is ready." Still no answer. My anxiety rose as the minutes turned into another hour with still no sign of him.

Finally, several hours later, at around eight o'clock, Luke answered when I phoned.

"Luke, where are you? Is everything okay?"

"Sure, Mom—I'm downtown, and I've met a bunch of people and we're having a great time!"

My bones softened, but I tried to sound calm. "Come on home now, Luke. Dinner is ready and we've rented a great movie for tonight." Without answering, Luke hung up.

Right then, all I wanted to do was hop in a taxi and ride through the city center looking for my son. Luke was an easy target for predators of all kinds—a vulnerable, at-risk young man with little sense of self-preservation or a clear lens through which he might sense danger. My logical brain told me to try to stay "in the moment," but my thoughts kept racing forward. I struggled to breathe deeply, trying every calming tactic I knew—and I prayed hard. Mark remained calm, at least outwardly, and I leaned on that.

About an hour later, Luke walked through the door, none the worse for his impetuous adventure—at least as far as I could tell. And fortunately, he never did that again. From that point on, we focused our energies on finding activities in the evenings and weekends to hold Luke's interest. We enrolled him in bass guitar lessons that required him to take mass transit, maneuvering his large, unwieldy guitar case in both directions. Thankfully, he always returned home on time and with the added benefit of a look of accomplishment on his face. We also hired a personal trainer, recommended by one of the staff members at the rehab program, to work with Luke two nights a week. He was good at his job, and Luke's confidence seemed to grow stronger along with his body. We were spending money left and right for his benefit, but at that point our only goal was to keep him safely occupied while he tried to learn strategies that would help him cope with his brain injury deficits. We viewed every cent spent on helping him as well worth it, but I kept wondering what we would do if those funds weren't available. It was a sobering thought, grounded in the realization that there were many families in just those circumstances. It had been a difficult enough road just finding a professional with sufficient knowledge to identify Luke's brain injury. How much more difficult would it be to locate social services organizations designed to help families affected by TBI?

Several weeks after the program began, Luke asked us if a fellow he had known from the town we'd just left could stay overnight at our apartment in the city. Before giving the okay, Mark asked some basic questions: Who is this guy? Do we know him? Luke was remarkably honest, and his answers shocked us.

"He's a homeless kid I met when I slept in the parking garage." He went on to say that this was a "good guy" who just needed some luck and opportunity.

Mark gave a guarded okay to Luke's request, with the right of refusal if we felt uncomfortable after meeting his guest. Luke seemed fine with that answer, and late that Sunday afternoon he brought his friend to the apartment. In his early twenties, the young man was polite, and he talked at length about the challenges he and his family had faced, and about his goals and how he was attempting to reach them. He seemed to be an honest young man down on his luck but working to change his circumstances, and when Mark and I spoke later, we realized we had both been touched not just by his story, but also by Luke's caring nature and his affinity for people in need.

We explained to both of them that since Luke had to attend classes the next day, his guest needed to leave when we left the apartment in the morning. He and Luke exchanged glances, and although the young man left with us as planned, something in those glances made me uneasy.

Luke's morning classes went okay, but when lunch break came, he told me he would not be returning for the afternoon sessions. Trying to stay calm, I suggested he first ask one of the counselors for permission to cut classes, as it was obvious Luke wanted to meet his out-of-town friend. I told Luke he should let his counselor know, and should be prepared to follow the counselor's directive. Luke, to his credit, did ask, and received a quick and emphatic *no*—but he left anyway. That was the Luke I had come to know in these past sixteen years—act first, think later, and make no connection between choice and consequence.

When Luke did not show up for classes after lunch that afternoon, the director was rightfully angry at our son's blatant disregard for program rules. He called Mark and me to a meeting and told us Luke was now "hanging by a thread" in the program, and if he didn't follow rules, he would be asked to leave. Despite my own anxiety about Luke's decision to cut classes, I could not believe my ears. After sixteen long and difficult years, we finally had the correct diagnosis and had been lucky enough to find a renowned program to help him with his specific needs. How could breaking rules not fit into the process of brain injury treatment, at least early on? Impulsive rule breaking seemed to be inherent to the condition, and I had an expectation that this program would teach Luke a better way to behave—not punish him for it. *How could the director expect Luke to completely reinvent himself after only a few weeks of initial treatment, and act as though he did not have a brain injury? Why would the threat of expulsion loom so quickly at the first sign of a poorly managed behavioral choice, which, I had already learned, is often an integral component of the behavior of those with brain injuries?*

That night, I couldn't sleep. I walked out into the street at two o'clock in the morning, not knowing where to turn and unable to settle my fears about Luke. For the first and only time in my life, thoughts of suicide bombarded my brain. I fought them off, but was startled and frightened by their uninvited presence. I knew Luke would act impulsively again. Unless the air he breathed in the rehab classes held some kind of magic, Luke would break rules again, and likely soon. With Luke now "hanging by a thread," the threat of expulsion awaited his next poor choice. This looming failure was even more confusing than those Luke had suffered prior to diagnosis. *Where would we turn then? What would happen to Luke?*

I felt devastated and frightened and lost. *What were we to do now?* We knew of no other options for our son.

"I Don't Know Why You're Here"

As part of standard procedure for new participants, the TBI director set up an appointment for Luke with a neurologist. When the doctor entered the examining room, he greeted us with a brusque and unexpected statement.

"I don't know why you're here." He squared his gaze at me and announced that Luke had no brain injury.

By now, I should have been braced for such remarks, but I was shocked yet again. Luke was a participant in a rehab center for people with brain injuries. He had undergone neuropsychological testing and had an MRI brain scan done as part of the program's entry process. Both tests identified Luke as having a TBI, as the SPECT scan previously had. *Why was a doctor now denying all this hard evidence?*

"I accidently dropped my daughter on her head when she was a few months old," he continued, "and she is perfectly fine. Your son does not have a brain injury."

Luke was in the room and couldn't have escaped hearing those words and their implications, unless by grace of the injury he hadn't processed them correctly. But the doctor's words were few and clearly stated, so Luke had likely taken the full brunt of their impact. Here was yet another professional denying the very injury that had been causing my precious son failure upon failure for as long as we could remember, but this time the denial came in spite of the tests and scans proving the injury. *Was there to be no end to this?*

The doctor gave Luke a cursory examination, and by the time we left his office, I was shaking with anger. I hoped Luke didn't notice my trembling hand as I pushed the button for the elevator; it wasn't his fault I was upset.

I went immediately to see the program codirector. To her credit, she was also rankled and quickly placed a call to the neurologist, who told her he had not had time to review Luke's records prior to our appointment. She emphatically asked him to find those records and take a good look at them. Later that day, I received an apologetic phone call from the doctor, and it was obvious that he had, by then, taken a close look at Luke's file. He confirmed the diagnosis, without doubt. *But at what cost to Luke?*

I related the apology to Luke as quickly as I could find him in a classroom. His demeanor had changed dramatically that morning after the appointment, and stopping the bleeding quickly was important. The codirector reinforced for Luke that he was exactly where he needed to be, and why, which seemed to help.

That good news from the program staff was complicated by their continued use of the phrase "hanging by a thread." I had hoped it would end once Luke's class-cutting incident was behind him, but it didn't. And each time they said it, which was weekly at least, my discontent and sense of foreboding grew stronger. Over so many years of having no answers for Luke, I had developed into a driven advocate for him, and that negative phrase caused me to bristle internally with anger and frustration. I felt a wedge forming between the program staff and me, my trust in them receding. I had to talk myself down from confronting their methods. I recalled what the director had said about Luke being unable to sustain another failure. If that were the case—and failing this program would certainly be a serious failure—then why was threat of imminent failure the constant message they chose to send him? I was confused and, in truth, angry with the staff because of it, and that would not help Luke's future there. I tried my best to put on at least a neutral, if not happy, face and to keep my complaints to a minimum, but my face mirrors my feelings all too often, and I likely showed my discomfort more than I realized.

Sometimes I wondered why the director bristled at me, until one day I recalled an early conversation between us. I had phoned him a few days after Luke's acceptance into the program to ask if it would be better for us to live in the city to lessen the cumulative effects of fatigue from commuting, and he told me it was fine for us to stay put and make that long hour-and-forty-minute journey twice a day, four days a week. On the first program day in September, the director learned we were now city dwellers. He displayed annoyance and, retrospectively, I guess he assumed I had chosen to disregard his advice. Mark had made the decision to move into the city, but the director didn't know that. Strike one. The director had also told me in the same conversation that addressing Luke's drug use could wait, and initially Mark and I intended to follow that directive. But when Luke went to camp and ran away while more than a thousand miles from home, panic entered into the mix and we made the mistake of sending him to a drug rehabilitation center. Strike two. It began to sink in that if Luke was "hanging by a thread," then I was at least partially to blame. *So punish me; help me to help him— but don't cut him loose. Please!*

My weekly meetings with Luke's assigned counselor were negative overall: Luke wasn't trying hard enough; if they were to invite him back for the next twenty-week session, he would need to work much harder. They wanted him to show enthusiasm for what he was learning, and they wanted him to have his shirt tucked in at all times and to sit up straight during all the presentations. They wanted him to look alive and to show interest while he worked on the repetitive efforts that would eventually build a new set of workable connections in his brain. All of those expectations seemed reasonable, but given Luke's long-entrenched bad habits, I feared they might be too high too soon. How could behavioral tendencies that had been misaligned for so long find so quick a resolution? I came to dread appointments with the counselor, and the way she would hold up her thumb and index finger to illustrate just how close Luke was to failing.

Whenever Luke and the other TBI participants were given feedback from the director and other counselors on their progress and on the program's expectations of them, they always received at least some positive reinforcement. In Luke's case, the staff members also made it clear that he had a lot of hard work ahead of him if he was going to form usable strategies to help him compensate for his traumatic brain injury deficits. As the weeks went on, the messages became increasingly less optimistic that Luke would find his way to success through the program. Although Mark and I noted huge improvements at home in Luke's ability to curb verbal outbursts, Luke's counselor discounted those observations. She made it clear that in her private sessions with Luke, she was advising him that he needed to work much harder if he were to be invited back to continue his rehabilitation. Backing Luke into a corner, elevating his anxiety level, made no sense to me. My confusion mounted with every passing week.

During one of my sessions with the counselor, I took a calculated risk. It was widely known among the program attendants that no questions were to be asked regarding the program's methods. Fearing for Luke's future well-being and fighting against a strong sense of intimidation, I asked the counselor how telling Luke he was "hanging by a thread" would help him. The director had clearly stated at enrollment that Luke could not withstand any more failures, and, from my perspective at least, that phrase was setting Luke up to fail. I knew I was out of my element: I had no formal training in brain injury rehabilitation. But I did have years of experience dealing with a child who had an undiagnosed injury. Through trial and error, I had learned the hard way some methods that helped and some that didn't, and feeding Luke negative messages was definitely on the "doesn't help" list. His best chances for positive outcomes came when he was treated with kindness, respect, and encouragement. Focus on what he was doing wrong, and he would fail every time. That much I had learned about my son.

When the counselor deflected my question about that intimidating phrase, I forged ahead and asked if they were taking into consideration the negative self-image Luke had developed over time from his repeated humiliations and failures. How were they intending to treat his accumulated psychological damage, or, more fundamentally, were they intending to directly treat that damage—or did they believe it would be repaired as a passive, ancillary benefit alongside behavioral and cognitive improvements?

I was desperate for answers by this point because, watching the program's methodology each day, it had become clear to me that it had a "one size fits all" design. Yet Mark and I recognized that Luke was not beginning his TBI rehabilitation on the same level as the other participants in the program. They all had memories of their lives prior to their brain injuries, and could draw from those pre-injury experiences to help themselves, with program guidance. Luke had no memories prior to his third birthday, so life with a brain injury was all he knew. How, then, could he be judged on the same playing field as the other participants? The director and his staff must have felt he could be helped by this one path treatment; otherwise, why would they have accepted him? Luke had begun this program with such hope. But as the weeks and threats of expulsion mounted, he sank lower into his chair every day in the cognitive training sessions, and some of the defiance that had accompanied his previous failures began to reappear. Mark and I spoke positively about the program to try to keep him on track, but that didn't seem to be helping.

Luke began to balk at the required business-casual dress code. For the men, that meant collared, long-sleeved shirts tucked into tailored, belted slacks. As a high school freshman, Luke had grumpily accepted even stricter standards (including a tie), so I had not anticipated a problem now. But here, as he was reminded at least weekly of his looming failure, he would often defiantly refuse to tuck in his shirt. A familiar recourse was emerging: Luke preferred to be seen as in control of his own defiance than to be viewed a failure in the classroom.

One day I asked the staff if they could recommend a good ancillary psychologist who could provide lateral help for Luke as an addendum to the program, but I was told that under no circumstances and at no time was I to take Luke for secondary psychological counseling. When I tried to ask why, arms went up in the "stop" position and heads shook "no" before my question could be completed. During lunch break that day, I took a walk with another of the mothers, whose son's frontal lobe brain injury at age eighteen manifested similarly to Luke's. I had heard her mention that she also wished for additional and supportive psychological help for her son outside of the program. I asked her if she had found someone and she immediately stopped walking and grabbed hold of my arm, turning me to face her. "Don't ask again," she said, teeth clenched. "And don't ask why. If you want Luke to be able to continue with his treatment, those are the rules. I tried pushing them and was threatened with expulsion. This is too important. Please, please just follow their rules. They're in place for a reason known to them, and we need to accept and let go of our own ways of doing things." I never understood the program's reasoning on that issue, but I was grateful for the reminder that it was my job to accept it because they were the professionals, and I was not.

The slow pace of progress and threats of expulsion were a far cry from our initial expectations when Luke began this program. My anticipation that he would need only a few weeks to learn reading skills had fallen by the wayside quickly, and the dream of him attending college and finding his way to becoming a successful physicist was by now completely dashed.

The pain of watching Luke lose hope day after day was unbearable, yet what was the alternative? He was already enrolled in this well-respected program, and he wanted rehabilitation for his brain injury.

The three of us needed to hold tight to the belief that he would find that path to freedom here, despite the bumpy start.

A Day at the Beach

Luke completed the first twenty weeks of the TBI rehabilitation program and, despite reminders that he was on shaky ground, he was finally invited to continue for another twenty weeks. The invitation, rife with warnings of looming failure if Luke didn't ramp up his efforts, was perhaps designed to inspire him to work harder, but it felt to me that the staff did not believe he would.

During the three-week break between sessions, we took a trip to California. Mark had a couple of business meetings there, and he asked if Luke and I would like to tag along, hoping to reward Luke for his efforts in the program and to encourage his continued progress.

While in southern California, Mark's client invited the three of us to play a round of golf with him. We spoke with Luke about the importance of maintaining decorum for his father's sake, and with trepidation, we accepted the offer. It was early in the trip, and Luke managed to ward off fatigue and impulsivity and pull it together for his dad. It was obvious from watching him that he was working hard to remain polite, and those attempts were succeeding even when his golf shots weren't. As Luke put into action some of the strategies he had already learned in the brain injury program, like taking deep breaths and silently counting to ten before reacting, he appeared confident in the process. The day went well.

We continued our drive up the gorgeous Pacific coast toward the second meeting in San Francisco, and were in for the treat of a lifetime when we arrived in the Monterey area. Mark threw the budget to the wind and arranged for the three of us to play golf on the famous Pebble

Beach course. From the first hole to the last, it was an experience to cherish. Luke smiled continuously, and we noticed how straight and tall he held himself. Playing golf at Pebble Beach was a dream come true for him. He was visibly tired after walking the course and after having worked hard to maintain composure during the previous few days, and agreed to take a long nap before dinner. The following day, we tacked on a whale-watching trip that he seemed to enjoy, despite indicators that fatigue was taking hold. Mark and I were impressed by how well Luke seemed to be doing, but we were not surprised when signs of a meltdown began to creep in. As we stood on the sidewalk after the boat ride, Luke cursed at me and spat on the ground for who knows what reason. His drooping right eyelid and slumped shoulders exposed his exhaustion.

The next day we were scheduled to travel the rest of the way to San Francisco for Mark's second business meeting. Luke asked if he could fly back home two days early instead of joining us. Because he seemed to have gained a semblance of self-control during this trip, however temporary, and because there were no signs of drug use but plenty of signals that he was worn out, we decided to take a chance and let Luke go home alone ahead of schedule.

We dropped him at the airport, praying for the best. As promised, Luke phoned us when he arrived back at the apartment, and I felt myself relax. There was a constant push-pull for me regarding Luke. I wanted him to have age-appropriate experiences, but knowing what was age-appropriate for him was not a straightforward process. Second-guessing was simply part of everyday life with Luke.

And a Night from Hell

Early in the second session of TBI rehab, Luke failed to come home one night after classes. I had not attended the program that day, so at first I assumed some of the participants had gone out afterward. Admittedly, that would have been unusual, but I didn't immediately fear the worst. Eventually, I tried Luke's cell phone, but it went directly to voice mail. Although his phone was always on, I rationalized that perhaps he had remembered to be polite in a theater or restaurant, applying strategies from the program.

An hour or so later, the phone rang; I ran to pick it up, certain it would be Luke. Instead, I heard an unfamiliar man's voice introducing himself as an attorney for one of the other TBI participants. Apparently, during lunch that day, some of the members had gone outside to smoke marijuana behind the classroom building and were spotted by a police officer. The others darted off, but Luke remained in place and was arrested for possession. He had used his one phone call from the jail to notify a program friend. That friend in turn phoned his attorney, who, as a parent himself, knew that we would be worried. He gained permission to provide us with the details of where Luke was being held, and told us that Luke's hearing was scheduled for midnight. I hope I was able to express my gratitude to this man despite my shock, but to this day, my only way of repaying him has been to pay it forward. What a remarkable gift he gave us.

I phoned Mark, and then practically ran to meet him at his office. We headed out to find the courthouse, in an area of the city unfamiliar

151

to us. After one transit transfer and a ride in the wrong direction, we finally located the building. A police officer at the entrance verified that Luke was being held there, but told us that we were not allowed to see him or speak with him. Then, likely recognizing we were frightened for our son, he smiled and suggested we have dinner and relax a bit, as the hearing was hours away. Not wanting to leave the area, we walked a few blocks, found a casual restaurant, dutifully ate a few bites, and then quickly returned to the courthouse. Knowing Luke was being held in a large city jail was about as frightening as anything we'd endured up to this point—somehow even more frightening than when he had disappeared for hours or days at a time.

Ever since Luke's behavior had begun to spiral downward, it had become increasingly apparent to me that unless something drastic occurred to help him, he would end up either homeless or in jail. I suffered from an almost irrational fear of either of those two things happening to him. The feeling that he was a babe in the woods had never left me, and had only been reinforced by the TBI program. We were taught that emotional maturity is mostly truncated at the age the brain injury occurs, which for Luke had been just shy of his third birthday. He had matured somewhat beyond that stage, of course, but he was well shy of normal for his age. Knowing that emotionally he was a small kid in a grown man's body and so vulnerable terrified me, as did the thought of him in jail or on the street—alone, hungry, and frightened. Just thinking about it now makes my stomach churn.

With hours to wait and anxiety rising, we ended up hiring an attorney already in the courthouse for another client. After looking into the details of Luke's case, he expressed concern that Luke had been caught with slightly more marijuana than would be considered a misdemeanor.

When Luke's case was called, the attorney explained that Luke was in the midst of receiving treatment for brain injury, and the judge gave him a one-year probationary sentence. The judge made it clear, however, that if Luke were to be arrested again at any time during the next 365 days, the judicial system would have no choice but to impose a mandatory jail sentence. Sitting in that courtroom awaiting the judge's ruling had taken me to the highest level of raw fear that I had ever felt, so it took a moment for the judge's ruling to sink in. Luke was free to leave.

Strangely, Luke seemed annoyed that Mark and I were in the courtroom, and he darted past us to leave the building on his own, manifesting the very emotional immaturity at the root of my angst. Thankfully, Mark was able to corral him and convince him to go back to the apartment with us. It was not easy to read Luke, and at this point, I was too tired and confused about the whole ordeal to try.

I struggled to contain my hurt over the fact that Luke hadn't called us after his arrest, and that he'd tried to run from us when he was set free. He had been pulling away from Mark and me since his failures had begun, as far back as middle school, but until this point I hadn't realized just how far apart we had grown. In so many ways, living with Luke was like living with an agitated, impulsive stranger whose next actions could not be predicted and, likely as not, would not be in anyone's best interest. I loved him and craved a relationship with him, but "relationship" implies a two-way connection, and ours seemed entirely one-directional. I was beginning to arrive at the heartbreaking realization that a close relationship with Luke might never redevelop.

Several days later, we learned that our insurance case manager had done her magic again and had secured insurance coverage for another twenty weeks of treatment. This was surprising news, and Mark and I were enormously relieved. But weeks later, on the heels of the news, the brain injury program, with quiet acquiescence from Luke, decided to end Luke's treatment, finally cutting that last thread that had held him in place. The director was quick to make clear the decision had nothing to do with the arrest, since self-medicating was not unusual within the brain-injured population. He repeated his contention that Luke hadn't tried hard enough, despite the behavioral improvements we had witnessed at home. I was confused and bereft, but Mark and I had no say in the decision.

The staff offered no options for us to consider—no other programs, no direction at all to keep some measure of hope alive. Just cool, quick goodbyes, and suddenly we were left to our own devices once again, despite my desperate request for guidance of some kind. We had sold our home in the suburbs, and were in the process of building one in another state, but it would be months before our lease expired and we could move out of the city and into our yet-unfinished new home. Without the structure of a brain injury rehabilitation program, and with the largest failure of all now under his belt, our fear was that Luke was at red-level risk of becoming a victim of impulsive bad decision-making. The chances of Luke avoiding another arrest while his brain injury remained untreated were slim to none. We had to find a safe haven for our son, one that might lead him out of his growing depression toward some kind of stability. And we had to find it soon, despite having capsized alongside Luke in a failure that could easily drown him, and us with him. Mark and I had to resurface quickly and fight for our son's life.

Abandoned

Over the years, I had tried to convince Luke that none of us is a victim. *Okay, I would say, you have ADHD* (and later, TBI), *but that doesn't have to stop you. You will learn ways around it. The important thing is to not give up.* But as I look back at this time in Luke's life, it is obvious he *was* a victim, and my words of encouragement, however well-intentioned, were far afield and more than likely a stumbling block for Luke. Mark and I needed guidance beyond basic parenting if we were to find a way to help our son.

Recalling the in-home interview Luke had with the dual-diagnosis residential TBI program director the previous summer, I traveled there to look at that program in earnest. While perhaps not as strong a cognitive program as the one Luke had just left, it looked like a good and viable option for the four months until our house was built, at which point we could consider outpatient alternatives in our new location. Luke reluctantly agreed to transfer to the residential program, and I took his agreement, reluctant or not, as indication that he still nourished a glimmer of hope for his future. He had always wanted to achieve, and his pluckiness to keep trying in spite of the obstacles in his way was remarkable. His early injury might have sidetracked his success, but it had not changed the natural spirit of the pre-injured boy.

Luke was assigned to a room in a separate one-story house within the facility, which he shared with three highly functioning residents. It was a wonderful setup for him, and the directors got him involved right away with classes on drug abuse and arranged to have him begin a community college program to learn auto mechanics. Luke loved cars, and the theory was this might give him his first taste of success. Automotive training was essentially hands-on, which cut down significantly on Luke's need to read.

Everything seemed to be going along fine for the first month or so, but then Luke was caught sneaking back into his room in the middle of the night. He had climbed out his bedroom window and walked two miles in drenching rain to a twenty-four-hour pharmacy to pick up cold medicines that would make him high. It is difficult to even write those words, since the thought of Luke in that untreated state of depression, feeling the need to so desperately medicate himself, saddens me to the core.

After this serious infraction of the rules, Luke was able to continue his classes, but he was moved to the "lockdown" building on the main campus. It was a much larger building than the smaller house he had to leave, and he shared that larger space with a host of other people, some of whose brain injuries and brain illnesses were far worse than his own. Mark and I knew it was for his own protection, but the conditions were pretty raw. We visited often, trying to reinforce that he had not been abandoned and that this was a short-term, temporary opportunity for him to learn strategies to help him cope with his brain injury without the use of drugs of any kind. When we visited, we hoped to see improvements in his demeanor and signs that he was making progress, but all we witnessed was his increasing anger and depression, manifested in his outbursts and in the poor care he was taking of himself. He stopped shaving, refused to get haircuts, and showered only occasionally.

Fourth of July weekend was fast approaching, and Luke became insistent that he and his friends from high school had made plans to spend the weekend together. He threatened to walk out of the program and hitchhike the ninety-minute ride back to his buddies, and the program director and Mark and I all knew he would do just that. He had impulsively run away from situations he disliked before, and he would almost certainly do it again. Against their better judgment, the program administrators made the decision to allow Luke to leave for those two days, provided I agreed to drive him there and bring him back again. I hated being put in that position, but agreed to their terms.

I spent a worried and uneasy few days in a hotel after dropping Luke at the home of one of his good friends (who was fortunately one of my favorites among them). I had no idea if he would be there when I went to pick him up in two days or not. But thankfully, he was, and despite his scraggly appearance, I heaved a huge sigh of relief as I watched him walk out the door and toward me.

I assumed Luke would be willing to comply with his treatment program for the two remaining months until we moved, fulfilling his end of the bargain, but when we arrived back at the facility, the counselors searched his bag and found a large amount of marijuana stashed in it and in his pockets. Again, a feeling of desperation set in. I was realizing Luke had, at the very least, an emotional dependence on marijuana that promised to compromise his treatment.

The program applied consequences to Luke's actions that day, but chose them carefully so they wouldn't interfere with his schooling. They wanted him to find and feel success, so he would want it and learn methods to keep it. When he wasn't attending automotive classes, he was required to participate in drug rehab classes and meetings. The hope for all of us was that those few months would be sufficient to break Luke from his drug use and set him on a path toward success.

Luke willingly attended the automotive classes, but he continued to spew words of hatred at Mark and me whenever we phoned or visited. He was obviously miserable at the facility, but he also desperately needed help. It's impossible to describe the sense of losing one's child while there is still life and breath in him, but that is exactly what it felt like. It seemed much of Luke's anger was a result of his TBI-related disconnect, due to which he often misunderstood our words or intent. The harder we tried to reach him and let him know how much we loved him, the more vehemently he acted out against us. The knowledge I had gained so far about brain injury was helpful in my efforts to understand Luke, but that was small consolation against the daily experience of our son seeing us as his enemy.

The residential program counselors had done thorough research into Luke's history at intake and learned that his fist-shaking episodes as a young child had finally been identified as seizures resulting from the brain injury. They decided to try to treat him with an anti-seizure medication, assuming it might calm some of his escalating outbursts. There had been some speculation among the staff of the previous program that those seizures had likely continued all along, invisible to the eye and remaining undetected.

Several days after initiating the new medication, however, the counselors called to report that Luke had smashed some furniture and was threatening more harm. The addition of the anti-seizure medication had been the only change to Luke's routine and, recalling how that same medication had caused a similar reaction in one of the other participants in the previous program, I asked them to stop giving it to Luke. Initially they refused my request and, over the next several days, Luke's condition worsened and his outbursts became intolerable. At that point I begged them to stop the medication, and with voiced annoyance and doubt, the counselors finally did. Thankfully, within a few days, Luke returned to his normal state of verbal-only outbursts. From that point on, they were as anxious for Luke to leave as Mark and I were. As luck would have it, our new house was finally complete.

Finding Our Way

I thought it would be easy.

I thought with a confirmed, documented diagnosis in hand, the process of finding help for Luke in our new location would be simple and straightforward. From our new state's Brain Injury Association I secured a list of three local brain injury specialists, all neuropsychologists, and scheduled an appointment with the first one for the week after the move. I tucked away the information on the other two, just in case, but I didn't expect to need it.

When we picked Luke up to take him to our new home, he walked out of the residential treatment facility building looking hopelessly lost, depressed, and unkempt, and he was foul-smelling and raging with anger. It was a long four-hour drive as Luke ranted ceaselessly, but I felt as though the worst in his life was finally over. I didn't try to stop his yelling or cursing, and held off telling him about the options for help in our new community. After a few days in our new home, though, with his anger reduced to a simmer, I approached him tentatively and told him about the scheduled appointment. I took a step back and waited a few seconds for his response, anticipating an outburst and feeling horrified that he held so much emotional control over me.

Once again, Luke surprised me by acquiescing and embracing another chance at help. That was the good news about his return to our household. Otherwise, he showered but didn't shave or wash his clothing or give any other indicators that he was stepping out of his state of depression. It was hard for me to look at Luke; I was so fearful of him becoming homeless and helpless on the streets one day if something didn't alter his course, and soon. He remained distant and disconnected from me, holding strong to his belief that we had abandoned him. I wanted so badly to put my arms around him and hug him tightly, as though I could embrace away his fears and depression and agitation and anxiety, and free him of the torment that showed so clearly on his face. He wouldn't let me near him, though, and I had no idea what to do except seek help for him as best I could.

Unfortunately, the first neuropsychologist didn't work out. He wanted Luke to engage in conversation and to look and sound as though he wanted to be helped. Normally a logical expectation, but Luke seemed incapable at that point of engaging with anyone, let alone someone he had just met and likely didn't yet trust. Memories of his recent stay at the residential treatment center held strong, and although he wanted help, Luke didn't seem to be able to "play along" until he found it.

Thankfully, he agreed to meet with the second neuropsychologist on the list also—but the same thing happened. The doctor's response sounded scripted: "You are disengaged, Luke. Here's my card. If you decide you do want help, give me a call and schedule another appointment."

I had Luke's HIPAA permission to sit in on these appointments and, not wanting to upset him, I had held back, contributing only a few words in answer to direct questions about Luke's medical, educational, and social history. But when this second dismissal was given, sounding almost identical to the first, I could no longer sit silent. "Is there any way, doctor, for you to treat Luke for depression now, so he can be able to engage and let you help him?" The doctor simply replied that Luke was an adult and could make his own choices.

But could he? Living with him, day in and day out, it hardly seemed possible. He was withdrawn, silent, not taking care of himself or his belongings, barely eating. But as an untrained parent, I still felt the pull to cede to professionals with more knowledge than I on the subject of brain injury. They each made it clear that I was to back away and allow

Luke to make his own choices. To give him more options, I found yet another neuropsychologist.

Luke agreed to see the third neuropsychologist. This time, we even left the house early enough to stop for a quick lunch. Although we ate in silence, there were no outbursts, and that felt like a step in the right direction. This time, Luke refused to sign the HIPAA form allowing Mark or me access to his medical chart. I pled with the doctor to make an exception under the circumstances of TBI, but his hands were tied, and he held his ground.

Following Luke's diagnosis eighteen months earlier, Mark and I had tried to secure a medical power of attorney so that I could act as Luke's designated agent and override the HIPAA regulations, but we were unsuccessful. Being over eighteen years of age when diagnosed and already an adult for legal purposes, Luke had to agree to it, and he didn't. The situation seemed ludicrous. We were blocked from helping our son, who was an adult by age only and who desperately needed help. It was a feeling of utter hopelessness and helplessness.

Every once in awhile, my thoughts returned to the diagnosing neurologist's words: "Oh, there's nothing to do. Your son's life is over. It is way too late for him." *Could this be? Why were we not able to find the help Luke so desperately needed—help that seemed at hand and viable? Why?*

One afternoon I closed my eyes and allowed myself the luxury of picturing Luke before and after the accident at the playground. One of my first memories was how concerned I had been that, even without obvious external evidence of injury, his face seemed changed, tormented somehow. He didn't look like the same child we had driven to the playground just hours before. His right eye drooped when he was tired; his sudden onset of anxiety and agitation was startling; and his furrowed brows remained painful to think about.

My thoughts drifted to an uncomfortable question: what would Luke's life have been like if, soon after the blow to his head, the brain injury had been identified? I imagined a life quite different from the one he was now living. I imagined that, with a timely diagnosis, Luke would have had immediate early educational intervention. By the time he entered kindergarten, a plan would have been in place to help identify any developing areas of cognitive difficulty (with the knowledge that TBI often carries delays), and his social difficulties would have been better understood and handled in a more effective, less scarring way. Luke would have been accustomed to a specialized educational plan from day one, and therefore likely would have been accepting of it throughout his years of schooling. His classmates also would likely have taken any educational interventions in stride, as simply something that Luke did differently. By this age, Luke would have had years of reading remediation, and might have even been happily enrolled in a college where educational interventions occurred routinely and were easily accepted and utilized. Luke's intelligence was intact and uninjured; with early and correct interventions, he could have been taught strategies to work around the processing issues that, undiagnosed, had derailed him.

I opened my eyes and shuddered, struck hard by the realization that none of what could have been done, had been done. Because of the sixteen-year delay in the diagnosis of Luke's brain injury, his situation was dire. Early intervention and help is possible and available for children with brain injuries. More is being learned every day, but without a diagnosis of injury, no help is offered. I wondered in that moment how many other children like Luke faced the same struggles that he did every day, simply because their brain injuries also remained undiagnosed and untreated.

Right then, I couldn't dwell in that thought. I needed to find a way to help my own son. He was teetering on the verge of an irrevocable despair.

In the weeks between appointments, Luke and I talked about continuing automotive classes in our new location. Despite his relentless anger about his stay in the residential facility, he had enjoyed those classes, and they provided a lifeline for setting up his future. I tried to engage him in the search for class options locally, but he slept all day, falling deeper and deeper into a pit of depression. Once again the task of deciding whether to let our son sink by putting him in charge of his own destiny, or to enable him to push forward toward a viable future, fell to Mark and me. Letting him drown was simply not an option. Basic parenting tools don't cover these situations, so we followed our gut instincts, dug in, and did the research for him. A promising community college option emerged, and once Luke visited the school and met the teachers, he was hooked. It was by now November, and despite missing the start of school in September, he agreed to enroll in classes beginning in early January. Mark and I were relieved, and we hoped this new door would provide the turnaround Luke needed. But meanwhile, Luke still needed help for his TBI impairments and his deepening depression.

The next lead we found was a former pediatrician turned ADHD specialist. Although he came highly recommended, I suspected that his area of expertise would no longer fit Luke's needs. This was a brain injury, not classic ADHD. My thoughts reverted to the ADHD psychiatrist from Luke's senior year in high school. When Luke had been diagnosed with TBI just months after seeing him, I had phoned that doctor to share the news.

To my surprise, the doctor responded, "Luke does not have a brain injury; he has ADHD."

"But Doctor, he does," I said. "I've seen the scans, and Luke has all the other criteria of a TBI."

I mentioned the spontaneous shaking of Luke's fists, which we now understood to have been seizures; Luke's failures to achieve academically in spite of a very high IQ; and his sudden behavioral and personality changes after being struck on the side of his head. The diagnosing neurologist had been clear in explaining that the ADHD similarities stemmed from the TBI.

Even with the evidence laid out for him, this otherwise kind and astute physician continued to deny TBI. I was becoming exhausted from what should have been the simple task of sharing information about Luke's diagnosis to try to unlock a path to a functional, satisfying, and independent future for my son. Instead, I still had to work hard to convince professionals that Luke had an injury, even after the brain scan had proven it. It was exasperating. We were getting nowhere.

Taking Luke to an ADHD specialist didn't make complete sense, given Luke's TBI diagnosis, but with no other options at hand, the appointment was made. Because Luke was enrolled in community college, this doctor prescribed a medication to help him focus, assuming that would help him learn. The ADHD medication Luke had tried in high school hadn't helped, but maybe another would.

When the new medication didn't immediately solve Luke's problems, this new doctor surmised that ADHD stemming from a brain injury might simply require a higher dose. But the third time he increased the dosage, Luke began to turn yellow. I phoned the doctor, who assured me that Luke was fine and that it was Luke's responsibility to report difficulties with the medication. There didn't seem to be anything I could do but watch and wait, and try talking some sense into Luke.

This high dose was having a serious effect, and Luke was clearly working hard to contain himself. He held onto the edges of the kitchen counter so tightly his fingers turned white; he ground his teeth; his eyes darted wildly.

A few days later, Luke stormed into the house wielding a steel-shafted golf club from the garage. His skin had turned a shade of deep orange and his eyes were wide and angry looking. Swinging the club in front of him, Luke threatened to smash the walls in our house. I had never before been afraid of my son. The provocation for this sudden, angry outburst remains a mystery to this day, but its escalation into threats of violence had a clear cause: the medication was making Luke very ill.

I dialed 911. We got Luke to the hospital, where the emergency room doctor managed to reduce the toxins in his body to a safer level, and was explicit in his instructions that Luke never take that medication again.

Acknowledging in the wake of that crisis that medication might not be the answer for Luke, the ADHD specialist referred us to yet another neuropsychologist—one who made house calls. After all we had been through thus far, hope might have been the one thing our family lacked. But hope runs deep, and somehow we again clung to the notion that maybe *this* time Luke would find the help he needed.

Following a two-hour in-home observation, the neuropsychologist made the following recommendations to the family gathered as a whole:

- Luke was to have thirty days to "get his act together" and conform to house rules;
- Luke, on his own and without reminders, was to handle assigned household chores; and
- Luke was to be respectful at all times.

If, at the end of the thirty-day period, Luke failed any of these conditions, Mark and I were to "put him and his belongings at the curb," letting him fend for himself until he "got it."

I looked over at Luke and watched the color drain from his face. He had apparently processed that message the way it was intended. Prior to Luke's TBI diagnosis being confirmed, I might have expected professional counseling to include a tough-love approach. But, having been injured as a toddler, Luke never had a chance to experience life successfully and to draw from his experiences. He did not make normal actions-to-consequences connections, and "hitting bottom" was a concept he would likely never conceptualize, unless and until he first received sufficient brain injury treatment.

This visit had been not only a waste of our time and money, but also an additional erosion of our languishing hope for Luke's future. More importantly, could this have caused even more harm to our son? Did he now think we actually would abandon him?

How long could this family hold onto hope? We were running out of options, but we still desperately needed to find help for Luke. The HIPAA regulations (and Luke's refusal to grant permission) were blocking our ability to help him through medical channels. And whenever Luke did agree to our inclusion, the people we found to help didn't seem to understand the daily challenges of his brain injury, or their recommendations were not targeted to help undo the ineffective habits he had honed prior to the diagnosis.

We decided instead to focus on supporting his efforts with the community college automotive classes and to secure job training for him. He seemed to enjoy attending the classes, in spite of the long ride to school each day. Because we hadn't needed a car when we lived in the city, Luke's driver's license had expired, and he had not shown interest in renewing it. So I drove him, and because the trip was almost an hour on an interstate highway each way, I generally stayed nearby and was always in the parking lot well before his last class ended. Luke could be so impulsive that he might easily hop into a classmate's car and head off somewhere. Catching him before he had a chance to be impetuous was key, and though controlling his life that way made both of us uncomfortable, the alternative was too hazardous to consider. I settled for trying to keep him safe. He endured those long rides with me without too much discontent and, fortunately, without too many outbursts. He mostly slept, and sleep was what he seemed to need most.

Luke became an ace student. His teachers liked and respected him, and he them. His life suddenly turned a corner when those classes began, and success began to build upon success. He even enrolled in summer classes, and over the course of a year, he maintained a 4.0 GPA and then aimed his long-range sights at a job with a high-end car manufacturer. He realized that would require an extra year of specialized training, but with Luke loving cars the way he did, the idea of more schooling didn't seem to deter him.

When Luke was a sophomore in high school, Mark, in an effort to encourage him to do better in school, had promised that he would buy Luke a car after he had completed two full semesters of college with passing grades. It took several months of periodic conversations between the two, and some pretty comic negotiations, before Mark settled on a price for this car, which was to be based on the GPA Luke earned during those semesters. They had even drawn up and signed an agreement that delineated a different price allowance for every possible GPA. Although these conversations had occurred before Luke's injury was identified, Mark wanted to use that "contract" now to build on his recent successes in the automotive program. Neither Mark nor I wanted Luke to drive if his brain injury would make him an unsafe driver, so we located a specialized driver's testing center at a nearby neuro-rehabilitation center. The center primarily served stroke survivors, but they were able to apply the same "driver-ready" principles to Luke's skills relative to his TBI. Mark told Luke that since he had earned top grades, if he received clearance to drive and then applied for a license, the two of them could go car shopping. Luke happily agreed, and he passed both the rehab and state tests easily enough.

Luke knew exactly which car he wanted and, with Mark's approval of the model, the two of them negotiated with the dealer to bring the cost down to Luke's allotted budget. A few days later, they came home with an adorable black compact with manual transmission—and Luke's face beamed. He took me for a ride around the neighborhood, and we shared a laugh about the Sunday afternoons we had spent when, at seventeen, Luke had tried to learn to drive a stick shift under my tutelage. "You will *feel* when you need to change gears, dear," I kept telling him, and he kept stalling the car. Finally, Mark took over the shifting lessons for one afternoon, and in short order they returned home. Luke marched into the kitchen looking for me, with a grin on his face. "Why didn't you tell me, Mom, that I shift when the _____ lines up with the _____?" He used the correct terms filling in those blanks, but they were foreign to me then and still are. With that memory in mind, I shared a rare and life-connecting laugh with Luke as he drove me around in his shiny new car, smoothly transitioning from one gear to the next.

Luke drove himself to school from then on, which was a huge release of my time. My driving responsibilities had left me little time to do much else. I was both physically and emotionally exhausted by then, but hadn't realized what a toll that routine was taking until my days suddenly became my own, and I could finally relax.

Luke was handling himself well with his new car, and he even took a few weekend trips to visit his high school friends who attended college several hours from us. He seemed to be managing both school and his social life with burgeoning temperance and care, and Mark and I began to wonder if the irritability he continued to display on the home front was perhaps a sign that he needed more independence. We tried everything we could think of to minimize those lingering outbursts, like supplying a small refrigerator in our TV room with his favorite prepared foods, and then leaving him alone in that corner of the house whenever he seemed to need it. Sometimes that worked, and other times we had to come up with alternative plans. But with the rest of Luke's life going well during this time, we focused most of our energies on encouraging his progress and trying to walk away from his emotional explosions.

Then, just as things were looking up for Luke, he learned that in order to graduate with an automotive certificate, he had to take several English classes and a social studies class—all of which required significant amounts of reading and writing. That news sent him into another downward spiral. Just when he thought he'd found a path to an independent and successful life, he realized his reading difficulties would likely once again derail him. The lack of a certificate would prevent him from obtaining the license he needed to find work.

Luke tried hard to continue with his schooling, even though the end result was now in question. Mark and I encouraged him to speak with his automotive teachers and to make an appointment with the dean. Luke wanted to handle this problem on his own, and we found his resolve encouraging. He dropped the ball, however, and never asked for help with his dilemma.

This was an abrupt and unanticipated turn in the road for Luke, and while his friends were making plans to graduate from college and begin their careers, he could see nothing in his future but a dead end. He still had another three or four semesters of automotive training before having to face the English and social studies courses that he felt would end in failure, and through sheer determination, he continued going to school.

But at home, the downward spiral continued. He began to leave on weekends more often, and he became more secretive and rebellious at every turn. The slightest request of him, like asking him to do his laundry or take out the garbage, caused him to roar obscenities at us. I rationalized that his amplified verbal outbursts were a direct result of his frustrations with those unexpected class requirements, and set out to find some way to help him face that problem head-on so he didn't feel the need to self-medicate, which I feared he was still doing. When I confronted him, he predictably raged, but in a calmer moment, he reminded me that marijuana was the only way he knew to quiet those perpetual noises in his brain. I hugged him and told him that, although I understood his logic, street drugs were not safe, were not legal, and were not allowed in our home. *But what would I be doing if I heard those constant sounds rattling through my own brain?* I felt like a hypocrite telling Luke to stay away from marijuana, when that might be the very thing he needed.

Soon another new option emerged: neurofeedback. When I first learned of it, I couldn't imagine how a few little wires attached to a person's head could help to retrain an injured brain. But Luke was willing to give it a try. His willingness was astonishing to me, given all the failures he had endured. I did a little research and was told by a neuropsychologist at a major medical center that this new technique was in fact quite successful, and that, if Luke did nothing else to help himself, he should do this. Unfortunately, Luke didn't notice immediate results and, after several months of weekly appointments, he gave up trying.

He perceived my pleas to continue those sessions as nagging, and that didn't help. I backed off and tried to figure out how to barter what little leverage we had left.

Without medical intervention, Luke's options were limited, and his success at school, though ongoing, was bringing him closer to what was perhaps an immovable roadblock. At home there were conflicts, as there are with any young adult living with parents. In Luke's case, though, his fatigue eroded his ability to restrain from the unbridled verbal attacks he had learned to curb at the first treatment program, through constant reminders and strategies from the brain injury rehabilitation staff. Without those professional reinforcements, our situation was unsustainable.

One Saturday afternoon, I called to Luke and he opened his bedroom door. As I reminded him to pick up his wet laundry from his bedroom carpet and come downstairs for dinner, his face took on a suddenly wild expression and his eyes darted angrily, never meeting my own. A moment later, something happened that changed the course of our lives. For the second time in two weeks, he shouted at me four of the worst words in the English language, a verbal onslaught I can't bear to repeat. All of a sudden, the years of frustration, angst, disbelief by professionals, and agony at witnessing my son's mounting failures and social isolation converged in a single moment, and my temper flared. I shouted back at Luke with such intense rage that even he looked startled. I was physically and emotionally spent and leaned into my meltdown. Never before had I felt so much anger at anyone, and as soon as the words left my lips and the anger volcano had spewed enough angst to return me to a rational state, I realized we were stuck in an eddy that would sap the life from all of us if we didn't alter our course. Something had to give. If it didn't, we would self-destruct.

Mark and I had been witnessing Luke's conflicted emotions whenever he returned home from visits with his high school friends, who were now graduating from college. His happiness for their success seemed matched by the disdain he felt for his own failures. Certainly, we thought, Luke's escalating outbursts were partially related to those conflicted feelings, so when that second major flare-up occurred, we decided a new direction might be to let Luke experience a more independent lifestyle, with us close at hand.

Luke was going to need to experience independent living while Mark and I were still around to help him with that transition anyway. *Was this the time to try?* We weren't going to live forever, especially under such constant stress, and it might take the remainder of our years to teach Luke how to handle life alone—how to plan and organize to pay his bills on time and keep food in his apartment, and how to know when food was too old to eat and when his clothes needed to be laundered and his apartment cleaned. We had, of course, been trying to work with Luke on all those tasks while he lived with us, but it was a constant battle, one Mark and I weren't winning. Luke's outbursts on the home front had reached such an intolerable state that we assumed a small degree of space would do wonders for all of us. We conjectured also that if Luke found success living independently, that might just breed more success. A win-win situation—or so we thought.

Success had to begin trumping failure if Luke were to survive and take control of his own life. He was doing great in school, but he had to face the looming social studies and English requirements and learn to advocate for himself in order to secure the help he needed to pass those courses. Once Luke was in charge of his own destiny, his achievements would start to build. I felt in my bones that Luke needed to pull away from us and that maintaining status quo would only impede his progress. Rationalization can be a wonderful short-term tool.

In stark contrast to my hopes, however, it turned out to be the worst decision we could have made. When we first suggested a separate living space for Luke, he balked and told us he was fine continuing to live in our house. I reminded him that his outbursts usually involved wanting to be left alone, and that an apartment—close to our house, but providing separate space—would give him a chance to be alone when he needed it. He even laughed a little when I told him I couldn't nag long-distance. Although not enthusiastic, Luke did not protest. Adapting to change had not been easy for him since early childhood, so we asked for his help in selecting the apartment, and then he agreed to go with me to shop for secondhand furniture.

Once Luke was in the apartment, however, his anger toward me escalated to a new level, though it seemed as much perseveration as rational anger. I had learned at one of the treatment programs that people with a brain injury will often hold one idea or thought in their heads indefinitely, beyond the limits of reason. Luke had demonstrated this throughout his young life in many and varied ways, so I recognized the signs. But having him continue to remain angry with me because he believed that I had abandoned him at the residential dual-diagnosis facility was, when emotion trumped reason, excruciatingly painful. Securing this apartment for Luke seemed to only fuel his perceptions of abandonment, and this was, for me, an unexpected development. My son felt discarded and frightened and alone—and I was unable to help him shake free of that feeling. Both of our hearts were aching, and there seemed to be no way to fix them so we could rebuild a relationship.

Falling Apart

While Luke was living in our home without professional help, Mark and I watched him slip from a vulnerable functionality into a behavioral abyss from which I could not imagine recovery.

The most frightening part for me was helplessly watching as Luke, physically grown but not emotionally or behaviorally equipped to handle adulthood, acted on impulse time and time again. He alienated everyone who loved him with abusive verbal outbursts. He manifested every imaginable sign of depression. His beard and hair were long and unkempt. He showed no sign of caring that his clothing was filthy, or that he smelled and seemed to lack any degree of personal pride. He would no longer play golf or tennis, despite his previous enjoyment of both games, and he withdrew to his room for hours on end. He even rejected an inexpensive jacket I bought for him (his had been stolen by a fellow resident at the previous treatment center) because it had a manufacturer's label sewn inside. It appeared he was rejecting any sense of connection to the functioning world at large, but in truth I had no idea how his thoughts were formed. I only knew they seemed foreign to me, and there was no road map to direct him to safety. He looked the picture of a young man with an unstable and very ill brain.

While attending the TBI treatment program, Luke described the confusion he felt about his failures, and how he had formulated the only plausible explanation for himself—that he was a "screwup." For someone who had wanted so badly to succeed to now find every path to success blocked was no doubt agonizing, and after many years of disappointments, I'm guessing Luke finally lost all manner of hope and human dignity.

Being unable to find a lifeline for Luke took its toll on all of us. Our little family grew increasingly desperate, and we each manifested that anguish in a different way. I tried putting myself in Luke's place and became overwhelmed with grief and frustration. I had learned enough about brain injury to realize that without some form of intervention or miracle, Luke would more than likely become homeless or end up in jail. I'd also learned that his TBI put him at a statistically high risk for suicide. Worrying about these things trapped me in a constant state of anxiety. Mark, a problem solver by nature, was unable to solve this most important of problems, and he withdrew and retreated into the safety and comfort of his books. Night after night, fear for my son's future kept me from sleeping. I worked hard to hide my raw disquietude from Mark, but my tears often jarred him from his own restless sleep, and we would lie in silence, having no words of consolation to offer each other.

Once Luke moved out of our house in January 2006, everything fell apart. His perception that the decision to set up an apartment for him was another act of abandonment held strong, and he became only more depressed. He agreed to meet with Mark at his office to pay bills once a month, but he refused to come to the house for dinner or even to watch a movie with us. Our hope that the separation would allow for a more relaxed opportunity to help impart life skills to Luke backfired. He maintained a defiant attitude, and refused my offers to take him grocery shopping or to come home for meals on the weekends. In fact, his anger toward me escalated to the point that he refused to speak with me at all. With Mark in the lead parental role, I backed off to give Luke space. The few times I did see him during the next ten months became failed attempts to learn from him what he needed, why he was so angry, and what we could do to help. I left voice messages several times a week just saying, "I love you, Luke." On his birthday in July, he agreed to let us take him out for dinner, but he shoveled the food into his mouth angrily and quickly, and he seemed jittery and anxious. Without engaging in conversation, he finished his meal and then leapt from his chair and asked to be taken back to his apartment. We obliged. As we drove away, my tears flowed uncontrollably.

Knowing what to do for our son was light-years beyond our parental abilities. We were learning that raising a child with a brain injury requires a group effort from family, friends, social workers, neuropsychologists, psychologists, neurologists, occupational therapists, and educators. To assume one or two parents or guardians can meet this challenge alone is unrealistic, and unfair to the child with the injury and to the family as a whole. Our child, now a legal adult, would likely remain an adolescent by maturity assessment. But we would not live indefinitely, and Luke needed to learn to take care of himself. *How would—how could—that happen?*

To try to address Luke's future needs in a practical sense, we contacted an attorney whose focus was special needs, and through her, we created a supplemental needs trust for Luke. The next step was defining its inner workings to ensure Luke would remain cared for during his lifetime— that he would continue to have a roof over his head, food in his pantry, access to medical care, and a means by which his bills would be paid. We located a bank in our state to act as trustee, and they assured us that once the trust became active upon Mark's and my death or disability, they would secure an outside agency to oversee Luke's basic needs. To secure the final requirement, one of our family members graciously agreed to supervise the practical care decisions being provided through the trustee bank several times a year. We were very grateful to her for agreeing to take on this small but important role in Luke's life.

In addition to the special needs trust document, we wanted to secure legal guardianship for Luke, recognizing that he would likely continue to need guidance and assistance throughout his lifetime. The attorney's response to our request floored us. Had Luke been diagnosed and the request made prior to his eighteenth birthday, the process would have been straightforward; however, because Luke was an adult for legal purposes, the court would provide him with his own attorney whose job would be to fight our request to limit Luke's personal rights, making us the "enemy" in Luke's eyes. Given Luke's history of running away when feeling frustrated or abandoned, our attorney strongly advised us to not take this legal action. The risk was too great, so we opted to keep doing what we were doing and pray for the best.

Meanwhile, Luke continued to meet with Mark several times each month to write checks to pay his bills, reinforcing that life skill. Mark gave him use of a low-limit credit card and, true to form, Luke was frugal with it. Fragments of hope for Luke's future remained, despite my unrelenting sadness that our relationship was effectively broken. I knew this was in part due to the perseveration from the TBI, which caused him to hold onto thoughts and not process them, but my awareness that Luke's injury was the basis of our painful detachment did not lessen the emotional pain of his rejection.

In late October 2006, Luke phoned our house early one evening. I was thrilled to hear his voice. He had locked himself out of his car, and he asked if I could pick him up. With our relationship in shreds, the optimist in me was delighted by his call. I hurried off to find him. Strangely, he hadn't wanted to tell me exactly where he was, and had provided only the landmark across the street from him as a directional guide. As I pulled into the parking lot my heart jumped with joy at the sight of him. His appearance was scraggly, to be sure, but that didn't matter. He was and always would be the joy of my life, and I so hoped at that moment that he had turned a corner toward forgiveness and that somehow, we could begin to repair our relationship.

Luke was carrying a brown bag that looked like it contained food, and he held a small book. As he climbed into my car, I looked beyond him and saw the building from which he'd emerged. It was a small community church, known for its outreach to people in need. My heart raced faster, and hope surged for the first time in a very long time. Luke seemed a little softer and kinder to me, but he refused my offer to come to the house and have dinner with us. As I drove into the apartment complex and slowed down, he opened the door and jumped out. I called after him as he ran away from me and, confused, I started to drive toward his apartment. He turned and yelled loudly at me to back off and leave him alone. I told him I wanted to wait until he got his spare key and take him back to his car, but he screamed "No!" and ran away.

Luke found a way to retrieve his locked car, and he did not reach out to me again. He returned to his pattern of ignoring my calls, and then he began to ignore Mark's. In early November 2006, he failed to show up to meet Mark for their routine bill paying. At the same time, Mark had begun to receive phone calls from Luke's automotive teachers, who were troubled because Luke had suddenly stopped attending classes. Concerned, Mark stopped by the apartment several times in the next couple of days but didn't find Luke there. When Mark finally reached him by phone, Luke assured his father all was well and that he would stop by Mark's office the following day to pay his bills. Mark waited and hoped, but Luke never came. Mark continued his attempts to reach him. But father and son never had an opportunity to speak again.

We had been taught at the first TBI program that without constant reminders, an injured brain can easily forget there is an injury and revert to unawareness that help is needed. Luke certainly seemed to be following this trajectory. Desperate, I found the name of an interventionist a few hours from home. We had a long conversation, during which he took Luke's history and said he would study the information and try to come up with a workable plan. He explained that, although Luke was self-medicating with drugs, this would not be a typical drug-related intervention. The interventionist would instead focus on reminding Luke that his difficulties stemmed from having a brain injury, and that he was in dire need of help for it. Realizing that Luke's situation was dire, he said he would devise a plan quickly and call back in just two days, on Friday, November 10. We made an appointment for a 4:00 p.m. phone conference that day.

Meanwhile, with Thanksgiving just around the corner, I increased my attempts to contact Luke by phone, happy that the holiday gave me an excuse to reach out to him, an excuse he might accept. But I left voice messages that remained unreturned, and then tried text messages. Luke would not respond.

I Love You, Luke

Friday, November 10, 2006

12:05 AM

As I made one last try for the night, Luke, much to my amazement, answered my call. We had a beautiful conversation. He sounded exceptionally tired, but also reflective. His anger seemed either diminished or worn out of him, and he promised he would see us on Thanksgiving, just two weeks later. Even the promise of a minimally renewed relationship with Luke thrilled my heart.

"I love you, Luke," I said, and the conversation ended.

3:15 PM

Luke drove his beloved car to the end of a secluded road and walked toward the trees, following the path into the woods and to his place of comfort. Knowing how he loved the calming stillness of water, I imagine that he took one long, last look at the river beyond the trees. Then, engulfed by despair, he lifted a gun to the injured side of his head, and pulled the trigger.

Suddenly, he lay silent and still, alone among the fallen leaves and the setting sun, at peace.

3:55 PM

Having arrived home half an hour earlier from an aimless afternoon walk around our little town, I tried to sit still and drink a cup of tea, searching for a sense of calm. Ordinarily, I would have completed my errands and been home by noon, but I'd felt particularly anxious and decided to stay out a while longer, hoping to settle my nerves with a bit of exercise and distraction. This was to be an important phone call and I had pinned my hopes on it, as I had done so many times before. *Please, please let this call matter*, I kept praying as I walked and breathed in the late fall air. Now, awaiting the scheduled call, I closed my eyes and willed myself to relax so that I could take in the interventionist's information with clarity of thought.

At exactly 4:00 PM, the phone rang as planned, but the news from the interventionist was not what I had hoped. In reviewing Luke's history, he realized that our two previous attempts to intervene and get help for Luke (first at the inpatient drug facility following high school graduation, and second at the inpatient TBI dual-diagnosis program) had not only failed but had backfired. He was concerned that another intervention, if only to raise renewed awareness for Luke of his injury and how much he needed outside help, was ill-advised and could easily cause him to run away again.

Instead, he asked if we would consider another type of appointment for Luke. He had in mind a psychiatrist whose dedicated work with people who had traumatic brain injuries had been remarkably successful. The interventionist realized the difficulty would be in eliciting Luke's cooperation, given the depth of his depression by this point, but he asked if Mark and I would be willing to take on that challenge and try to get Luke to the appointment. Of course we would, I told him, and thanked him for his insight and for this lead. He told me he would quickly arrange an appointment for us, and would call first thing Monday morning. As we ended our conversation, I shuddered, the offer of hope and help clouded by a strong sense of foreboding.

I had no idea that, at that moment, my son was lying dead in the woods, not a mile from our home and lost to us forever, having put an end to his nineteen-year struggle to find help. He had lived until he no longer could, until the realities of his long-undiagnosed and untreated brain injury left him bereft of the one resource that had kept him with us until now: hope.

A small Bible was found in his apartment, along with paperwork indicating a renewed interest in finding peace through God's love. That knowledge has allowed me some sense of comfort, and I have no doubt that Luke lives now among the angels, enjoying an eternity of love and peace.

Godspeed, Luke. I love you.

Epilogue

I believe my son's story ended tragically for one reason only: his brain injury remained unidentified and untreated for most of his twenty-two years.

I believe that the professionals whom we encountered along the way, with few exceptions, cared for Luke and did their best to help him. These were consummate professionals, skilled in their crafts, and remarkably good at their jobs outside of brain injury. I have chosen not to name or identify them in any way because, in my opinion, they should not be the focus of Luke's story. They did the best they could with the knowledge they had at hand. The issue is the need for increased awareness, so to maintain that focus, I have chosen to use pseudonyms throughout.

Since Luke's death, however, I have encountered a few professionals, well trained in identifying brain injury and in a position to make an influential difference, whose messages have thoroughly discounted the observations and feedback of parents of brain-injured children. In one instance, I participated as an invited member of a large panel that included neuropsychologists and neurosurgeons as well as educators, family physicians, and some other parents whose children had been affected by brain injury. We were all given assignments to present, but each time it was my turn to speak, the moderator, a neuropsychologist, waved her hand to bypass me. On another occasion, I was invited to sit in on presentations about TBI by a panel of highly respected doctors and researchers. One of the speakers listed criteria considered important in assessing the possibility of a head injury in an emergency room setting.

I was exhilarated by the information, realizing how application of it could help so many whose TBIs might otherwise remain unidentified. Then, on the next slide of his presentation, he listed criteria that should be ignored in making that same assessment. The first item to ignore, he said, was parental observation. I began to tremble, feeling suddenly assaulted. The effect of that comment was visceral for me.

Who better than a parent to recognize the very changes in a child that might lead to injury identification? Wouldn't identifying brain injury be better served through collaborative efforts than through exclusion? I might not be a physician, but I was certainly able to identify changes in my son that might have led to the correct diagnosis. *Who better to know the child than the parent?*

According to the Centers for Disease Control (CDC), acquired brain injury continues to be the leading cause of death and disability among children. If that is the case—and statistics clearly show that it is—why then is it still so poorly understood and recognized? This gap between statistics and practical understanding and diagnosis is the sole reason I have told Luke's story. Here was a little boy whose blow to the head was witnessed and who changed suddenly and dramatically following his accident. But, because there was no outward sign of injury and because the changes in him were more behavioral than physical, medical and educational professionals ruled out the possibility of brain injury. So Luke remained undiagnosed, misunderstood, and without treatment or targeted help of any kind. Society blamed him, as though he were choosing to fail. He didn't ask for help because he didn't know what he needed. He eventually absorbed the message that he was somehow causing his own difficulties, and when failure overwhelmed him, as it inevitably would under the circumstances, he simply let go of living.

My goal, and I hope yours as well, is to ensure that Luke's story will help to raise sufficient awareness about brain injury that his story will never again be repeated. The good news is that your family's story, your patient's story, or your student's story can have a much happier ending, as awareness of traumatic brain injury grows, along with a better understanding of what TBI means and how it develops.

If, as you read Luke's story, you recognized your brother, your uncle, your patient, your student, your niece, your mother, your child, or even yourself—what can you do?

Plenty.

First, trust your instincts.

If you are having cognitive difficulties that can't be explained and have not been diagnosed, or if the diagnosis you received doesn't fully define what you are experiencing, is there a chance you have sustained a brain injury? Do you recall being struck on the head at any time in your life, when you were either unconscious, or dazed and confused, for a time afterward? If so, did it cause you to feel highly agitated and/or anxious, or affect your memory or your ability to process information? Did your symptoms linger? Have you been having difficulty succeeding at school or at work since that time? If so, a thorough examination by a brain injury specialist might be helpful to either confirm or eliminate the possibility that your symptoms are the result of a traumatic brain injury.

If you are concerned about a family member or close friend, please talk with that person and ask if an event occurred involving a blow to the head. If it is your child, try to recall any incident that might have resulted in a head injury, like a fall from the monkey bars at the playground, or a strike to the head with a baseball or bat during a game. If nothing comes to mind, ask your nanny or babysitter if they can recall an accident involving a blow to the head, even if it did not result in an open wound. A fall down some stairs, maybe; or a tumble from the jungle gym or slide at the park. Do you recall a sudden change of behavior, especially involving agitation and anxiety? If so, can you think of anything that might have precipitated those sudden but lasting changes in behavior? A car accident, perhaps? Or your baby being shaken in any way? Was domestic abuse a factor? I am neither a medical nor educational professional, but I have learned since Luke's injury was diagnosed that there are many causes of brain injury, and that there remains a less than complete awareness among professionals of how it happens and what it looks like when it does occur. Information you may have, like recalling an incident when a blow to the head occurred, can be helpful when shared with a medical or educational professional.

Next, connect with resources. I've compiled a short list to get you started; there are now, fortunately, many options available. Knowledge about the brain is expanding in leaps and bounds, so the process of finding help will hopefully become easier in the months and years to come. Please know that it might take several tries before finding someone who believes you, even with information and awareness about brain injury coming to the forefront through the efforts of sports teams and the military. Judging from my own experiences and the experiences of families who have contacted me since Luke's death, however, general childhood injuries that are unrelated to sports or military service can more easily fall through the cracks and remain unidentified and undiagnosed, as Luke's was.

With your help, it is my hope that all childhood TBI will soon be quickly and effectively identified, giving every affected child the opportunity to reach his or her potential, with the added benefits of acceptance and understanding.

Finally, speak up. Speak often. Let your concerns be known—to your doctor, the pediatrician, classroom teachers, the school principal, legislators, family members, and friends. Because pediatric traumatic brain injury remains poorly understood and recognized, it often results in social isolation and self-doubt that can carry into adulthood. Learn all you can, trust your instincts, and then plead for help to any medical or educational professional who will listen. Contact your legislators to mandate change in what is being taught to students of medicine and education. If no one listens or takes your concerns seriously, try again. Keep trying until someone finally does pay attention.

If you are a medical professional, a psychologist, or an educator, I hope you'll read Luke's story carefully to learn more about what TBI can look like and how easily it can remain unidentified in children, or in adults who suffered TBI in childhood but who continue to struggle because they are not yet diagnosed. The professionals whom we encountered were not bad people; they simply had not been trained to identify traumatic brain injury, particularly the closed-head variety Luke suffered. Please take it upon yourselves to learn more than you might have been taught. Many families are counting on you to help them.

If you are a legislator, please work to broaden HIPAA regulations to allow access of medical information to caregivers, whose hands are tied without it. Please expand required textbook minimums to include more information about childhood TBI and how to identify it. Please work to bolster programs and funding for people with traumatic brain injury. Costs are prohibitively high, even for diagnostic purposes, and services far too limited. My fear that Luke would end up either on the street or in prison after we were no longer alive to watch over him is more than likely a common fear among affected families.

If I had it to do over again, I would have stood in front of the pediatrician, the pediatric neurologists, psychologists, and Luke's teachers as many times as it took to make them believe me. I didn't know enough about brain injury then, but I know now. And, hopefully, by learning from our experience, so do you.

If our lives are just stones across the water, I want Luke's ripples to go far. I want them to touch the lives of other children and adults like him who suffer from TBI and struggle to live functional, fulfilling lives without self-blame, and with a belief in good things to come. I hope that by sharing Luke's story, you, your patients, your students, your constituents, and your loved ones will find the help they need so their stories can have happier endings. Thank you for whatever you can do to help.

List of Brain Injury Resources

- Brain Injury Association of America (BIAA), www.biausa.org, 1-800-444-6443

- Brain Injury Research Center (BIRC), www.tbicentral.org, 1-888-241-5152

- BrainLine, www.brainline.org, 1-703-998-2020

- Traumatic Brain Injury National Data and Statistics Center, www.tbindsc.org

- Brain Trauma Foundation, www.braintrauma.org, 1-212-772-0608

- National Center for Injury Prevention and Control, www.cdc.gov/ncipc/tbi/TBI.htm, 1-800-232-4636

- National Institute of Neurological Disorders and Stroke, www.ninds.nih.gov/disorders/tbi/tbi.htm, 1-800-352-9424

- The Perspectives Network, www.tbi.org

- Brain Injury Home, www.tbihome.org

- Brain Injury Resource Center, www.headinjury.com/resources.htm, 206-621-8558

Acknowledgements

Poring over these memories of Luke was a difficult process, and without the insights, encouragement, and help of many people, *A Call to Mind* would have likely never been completed.

My first debt of gratitude is to my husband, Mark, whom I love with all my heart. His enduring support and patience throughout this endeavor have meant the world to me and, whenever I was about to quit, he encouraged me to see the project through to completion.

Loving appreciation goes to three darling nieces: Susan Haas and Kris Golden, who are elementary school teachers, for helping to stir my efforts to begin a TBI awareness campaign; and Karen Krickus, whose beautiful creativity designed and launched my previous advocacy endeavors. I love you all dearly.

Next, much appreciation goes to Dr. Wayne Gordon of Mount Sinai Department of Rehabilitation Medicine in New York. I met Dr. Gordon after Luke died, but he took hold of Luke's story and initiated an awareness video of it that he sent to medical schools in the US for tutorial use. He then assigned to me the task of writing this book, helping me to work through the pain in the process. And to Dr. Margaret Brown, whose edits of the video and advocacy endeavors were invaluable, for her guidance and her friendship. Many thanks to you both.

A big thank you also to:

Lucinda Bartley, whose hard work and perseverance led me to a better understanding of how to write a book;

Dr. Lori Korinek for her annual invitation to tell Luke's story to her graduate students of education at the College of William and Mary, which has led to a cherished friendship;

Patrick Donohue, whose daughter Sarah Jane was brutally shaken as an infant, for embracing Luke's story and for his tireless efforts on behalf of children with TBI;

Everyone at Brandylane Publishers, especially to Robert Pruett and Tamurlaine Melby, an enormous thank you for believing in and taking such wonderful care of Luke's story, for your insightful editing and for the beautiful end product.

Finally, a loving heap of gratitude to the friends and family who understood and whose support and encouragement kept me going as I tackled this project, when at times all I wanted to do was put these memories on a shelf and leave them there.

About the Author

Claire Galloway has been advocating for greater awareness of closed-head traumatic brain injury in children since 2008. She has spoken at several brain injury conferences and to students of education. This is her first book. She resides in Virginia with her husband Mark.

CPSIA information can be obtained
at www.ICGtesting.com
Printed in the USA
FFOW02n2344100118
44429997-44188FF

9 781939 930941